The Healing Power of Acupuncture

The Healing Power of Acupuncture

Michael Nightingale

JAVELIN BOOKS
POOLE · NEW YORK · SYDNEY

First published in the UK 1986 by Javelin Books,
Link House, West Street, Poole, Dorset BH15 1LL

Copyright © 1986 Michael Nightingale

Distributed in the United States by
Sterling Publishing Co., Inc.,
2 Park Avenue, New York, NY 10016

Distributed in Australia by
Capricorn Link (Australia) Pty Ltd,
PO Box 665, Lane Cove, NSW 2066

British Library Cataloguing in Publication Data

Nightingale, Michael
  The healing power of acupuncture.
  1. Acupuncture
  I. Title
  615.8'92   RM184

  ISBN 0-7137-1716-5

Typeset by Word Perfect 99 Ltd, Bournemouth, Dorset

Printed in Great Britain by The Guernsey Press Co. Ltd., C.I.

Contents

Foreword

Today, to unmask the mystery of acupuncture meridian theory has become a key problem in acupuncture as well as in other traditional medicines. This is because the rapid development of various methods and the discovery of phenomena in natural medicines obliges us to explain the basis of the meridian system in scientific terms.

In fact, encouraging progress has been made in the last decade. Through different paths, doctors and scientists have proved that the meridian system is not only a universal sensory phenomenon, but that it can be verified by a variety of physiological experiments using the electromyogram, the electroencephalogram etc, and biophysical techniques involving acoustic, photo, thermal and electrical techniques as well as nucleo-physical methods. The meridian does really exist.

It hardly needs saying that we still have a long way to go and much to do. However, under the guidance of the philosophy and principles of traditional Chinese medicine, and grasping tightly the meridian phenomena it is hoped to solve the meridian system with all the advantages of modern technology involved in biophysics, biochemistry, molecular biology, biological engineering, modern morphology, etc.

To accomplish such a project doctors and scientists must be dedicated to the modernisation of the traditional acupuncture clinic! We commend *The Healing Power of Acupuncture* by Professor Nightingale, in which he has expounded some of the recent scientific progress in our attempt to fully explain acupuncture and yet at the same time has welded this into the solid framework of traditional Chinese medicine.

Zhu Zong Xiang
Professor of Biophysics
Institute of Biophysics
Chinese Academy of Sciences
Beijing
1986.04.28.

Introduction

Acupuncture has been a popular form of treatment in the Orient for over 4,000 years and it is almost certainly one of the oldest methods employed by medicine. Whatever its exact origins, acupuncture quickly became a major resource of Eastern healers, and so it remains today – China claims a million registered acupuncturists and Japan 50,000.

In the past doctors in the West found it difficult to believe in the efficacy of acupuncture because it didn't fit in with their traditional concepts about the anatomy and working of the human body. They couldn't accept that diseases could be diagnosed by feeling twelve distinct pulses at the wrist or that the sum total of human illness was due to an imbalance between the opposing life forces of the *yin* and *yang*. Likewise, they found it impossible to place any special significance in the named acupuncture points, and couldn't believe in the idea of the circulation of *qi* energy along the twelve meridians or pathways which acupuncturists believe run up and down the body on either side. Nevertheless, they were forced to concede that acupuncture could, and very often did, relieve pain.

In recent years the West has taken a far greater interest in this ancient form of healing and today acupuncture is practised all over the world. However, surgery under acupuncture analgesia, which has been much researched, has scarcely been done outside China and Sri Lanka. Similarly, much of the real achievement and potential of acupuncture still remains obscure to the majority of people, including doctors.

Nowadays there is much less scepticism even among the medical profession. Research by a team of doctors at St Bartholomew's Hospital, London, in 1981, into the use of acupuncture in the treatment of chronic back pain, reported a cure rate of 70-75%. Similar results were obtained by the UK Consumers' Association when research was carried out, in 1972, among members who had visited an acupuncturist for lumbago, sciatica or non-specified rheumatism, for which doctors had given pain-killing drugs – 70 per cent were relieved of their pain. As Dr Andrew Stanway observes in his book *Alternative Medicine*, 'most people who go to acupuncturists are the hopeless cases that orthodox medicine can't cure – yet 70 per cent of them improve. This is remarkable by any standards.'

To many people it seems that modern scientific medicine, for all its accumulated learning and vast financial resources, has failed to provide the necessary guidance as to how they should live to prevent ill health, nor has it provided a cure for a large number of their illnesses. Advanced surgery may give the impression of medical and technological mastery of health problems, yet the unpalatable truth is that most operations could be avoided. Some of the many conditions for which there is no medical therapy or where it is only possible to ease the symptoms with drugs are as follows: arthritis, asthma, back pain, bronchitis, chickenpox, the common cold, many types of depression, eczema, German measles, hay fever, many forms of heart disease, hepatitis, herpes, influenza, measles, migraine, multiple sclerosis, muscular dystrophy, Parkinsonism, sciatica, sinusitis and numerous ill-defined problems. In the case of a few other illnesses, such as some forms of cancer, the treatment can be so severe and disturbing that patients have seriously wondered if the treatment is not worse than the disease. Moreover, the state of our health bears little relationship to the ever-increasing expenditure devoted to medical research and treatment.

It is difficult to assess the negative results of drug therapy but in the USA in 1970 it was estimated that the cost of complications caused by medically prescribed drugs was in excess of a billion dollars! This takes no account of loss of life and incapacitation and, when it is realised that more people are killed each year in the USA and the UK by prescribed drugs than by accidents on the roads, it becomes obvious that we should no longer remain complacent about the frightful expense in human terms of modern drug therapy.

There is an old Oriental saying that if you give a man a fish he will eat for a day, but if you teach him to fish he will eat every day. This applies to medicine: if you give a treatment which relieves symptoms you help the patient temporarily but if you teach a person how to live correctly he will remain healthy and have no need of treatment. Clearly, we need an all-embracing system of medicine which can dispense powerful drugs when necessary, but which can also address itself to health problems with simple, non-toxic measures which also promote general health rather than suppress unpleasant clinical symptoms. Acupuncture and Traditional Chinese Medicine not only effectively treat most illnesses safely and without adverse effects but also enhance health and act as preventive systems of health care.

In addition, for those prepared to change their life-styles, Traditional Chinese Medicine clearly points the way to correct living in conformity with the laws of nature. For those who do not wish to make such changes or who are unable to accept the value of doing so, acupuncture still remains a powerful treatment when things do go wrong, without the harmful effects of drugs. Of course, this only applies to the practice of acupuncture by properly qualified practitioners and it is the firm belief of the author that acupuncturists should also be qualified in orthodox medicine. The medical profession needs to recognise, however, that all properly trained specialists such as osteopaths, chiropractors, homoeopaths, medical herbalists and, to a large extent, physiotherapists do have adequate medical training which fits them ideally to learn and practise acupuncture. Once this is accepted a way could perhaps be found to unite medical practitioners and put an end to such terms as 'alternative medicine' and 'complementary medicine' which are misleading and counterproductive.

To the acupuncturist healing is something that transcends treatment and is difficult to analyse in a scientific manner. It is in healing where much of the *art* of medicine resides. Acupuncture promotes healing by its ability to harmonise the vital forces, regulate body functions and balance the emotions. Nevertheless, it cannot be successful unless the patient helps himself by regulating his own life, enhancing his vital energy and balancing his emotions. Whether the patient's prescription is a pharmaceutical drug, a herbal or homoeopathic remedy or an acupuncture needle, unless he is willing to take responsibility for his own health he will never be doing what is best for himself. It is the task of all physicians of whatever persuasion to assist their patients in this process and in so far as they do that they are true servants of their patients.

It is hoped that this book will assist people to become more conscious of their own ability to deal with their health problems and, if it does, that will be the reward for having written it. If readers also learn about acupuncture this will be considered a bonus.

1 *The Acupuncture Renaissance and the Ancient Tradition*

In the summer of 1984 a young man suffering from an acute and severe attack of bronchial asthma arrived for treatment at the Acupuncture Department of the South Colombo Hospital in Sri Lanka. The medical treatment which he had previously undergone, including steroids, had been a complete failure and, having heard from friends that patients with asthma had recovered after acupuncture, he had just begun a course of treatment. He willingly obeyed the injunction of the consultant who, contrary to normal medical advice, instructed him to stop his steroids – a course of action which had been taken many times before with successful outcome. With his sound training and experience in Western medicine coupled with a vast knowledge of acupuncture, this consultant was one of the few doctors brave enough to contemplate such drastic management of a patient. Now, with his customary deftness, he placed an acupuncture needle in a point found just at the top of the patient's breast bone and enjoined a group of Western doctors visiting his clinic to wait a few minutes and watch carefully. To their amazement, the patient's breathing had almost returned to normal within five minutes. The patient continued with daily treatments for a couple of weeks, after which time he reported that he was entirely free from asthmatic attacks and his visits to the hospital were slowly phased out.

This story may sound surprising, yet it relates a commonplace event at the Colombo hospital. Similar stories could be reported from acupuncture clinics the world over, although the precise sequence of events may differ and the period of being weaned off Western medical drugs would normally be much more protracted.

A few years previously, in the same hospital, surgical operations – including the removal of wombs, their repair, hernias and the removals of tumours – were being performed several times per week under acupuncture analgesia, and many of these were witnessed by the author. In fact, the largest parotid tumour on record was removed from a man in Sri Lanka under acupuncture and a few hours later the patient was sitting up in bed sipping tea and chatting with us – a remarkable event by any estimation.

THE ORIGINS OF CHINESE MEDICINE

The use of a sharp instrument to pierce the skin at certain strategic points was a medical treatment practised at the dawn of history. Over a period of time a highly sophisticated form of medicine had evolved in China which incorporated this procedure, together with moxibustion (burning a piece of dried herb over the point), herbal medicine, massage and dietary regulation. The term acupuncture is itself a very much more recent word and was probably derived from the Latin words *acus* (a needle) and *punctum* (particle of the verb 'pungere': to prick), although the early practice was almost certainly carried out with pieces of flint, bamboo or bone. Later, gold and silver needles were manufactured and these were used to treat the nobility. When, in more recent times, needles were made of stainless steel, some authorities regarded these as inferior to gold and silver, but experience all over the world with stainless steel needles has shown that these are the best type of needle for most purposes in acupuncture.

As acupuncture is such an ancient art, its origins are to a large extent shrouded in mystery and legend. The three legendary Emperors Fu-Hsi, Shen Nung and Huang Ti are generally regarded as being the originators of Traditional Chinese Medicine. Fu-Hsi is sometimes called the Adam of China and is said to have taught that the cosmos is divided into two complementary, interacting parts known as *yin* and *yang*. Since this concept forms a vital foundation to the entire philosophy of Traditional Chinese Medicine it will be examined more closely in the next chapter. Shen Nung, who lived around the year 2700 BC, is regarded as the Father of Chinese medicine and is said to have formulated the idea of acupuncture. He also invented the plough and is regarded as the greatest figure in ancient China. Huang Ti (*c.* 2697-2599 BC) is known as the Yellow Emperor and is supposed to have begun the construction of the Great Wall. He is supposed to be the author of the *Nei Jing* – 'The Yellow Emperor's Classic of Internal Medicine' – which is the earliest book on acupuncture still existing and is regarded as the canon of Traditional Chinese Medicine. It is probable that the collective work, based upon the sayings of the Emperor, may have been compiled around the third century BC and antedated to enhance its authenticity. In the first part we are entertained to a dialogue between the Emperor and his Chief Minister and physician, Ch'i Po, describing their view of human physiology, the origins of disease and how these should be treated. The importance of conforming with the laws of the universe is stressed and it is interesting to note that at the beginning of the book Ch'i Po tells his readers that 'In ancient times people patterned themselves upon the *yin* and *yang* and lived in harmony.' He writes of harmony, temperance in eating and drinking, regular hours for sleeping and rising and life extending for a hundred years. 'Nowadays,' he remonstrates, 'people are not like this; they use wine as beverage and they adopt recklessness as usual behaviour.' He goes on to say how they make love when intoxicated, dissipate their vital forces in passion, are discontented and seek amusement of the mind and do not keep regular hours. All this causes them to degenerate after the age of fifty! Have times changed at all, we might well ask?

It is also interesting to note that the author of the *Nei Jing* anticipated William Harvey who first expounded the theory of the circulation of the blood in the West in the seventeenth century AD. More than 4,000 years earlier Huang Ti wrote 'The blood is under the control of the heart, the heart is in accord with the pulse. The pulse regulates all the blood and the blood current flows in a continuous circle and never stops.' Apart from its teaching about the circulation of the blood, the *Nei Jing* also describes some fifty different types of pulses and thirty-seven different kinds of tongues: both are aspects of diagnosis which have consistently occupied a most prominent position in Traditional Chinese Medicine. It also relates how adverse climatic conditions and harmful emotions such as anger, hatred, jealousy, fear, worry and anxiety are the causes of disease: important facts which Western medicine is just beginning to discover!

THE SPECIAL NATURE OF CHINESE MEDICINE

What is unique about Chinese traditional medicine is that it provides us with a complete explanation of how the body works, how the vital forces are formed and how they may become unbalanced. Above all, it views the human body as a vital whole, infused with energy, which is more than the sum of the workings of its various organs. This, of course, is unlike the more mechanical view of Western medicine which sees the organism in purely physical terms. The same thinking was applied to other branches of science and, although some of their ideas may sound a little quaint to modern ears and some of their theories a little picturesque to Western scientists, we are all well advised to consider them and not simply to discard them out of hand as fairy tales.

MAN AS A MINIATURE UNIVERSE

One of the greatest stumbling blocks encountered by Westerners when studying acupuncture is caused by their failure to realise that it is based upon concepts which are still somewhat obscure to us. For example, it sees man as a miniature universe – a microcosm within the macrocosm. The microcosm reflects the macrocosm and is subject to the same laws. Moreover, it also affects the macrocosm in rather the same way that each individual member of society affects society as a whole. The course of nature is guided by the *Tao* – the unknowable which becomes expressed in the formation of the dual forces *yin* and *yang*. It is the *Tao* that brings about the ever recurring changes, such as day to night, the waxing and waning of the moon, light to dark, the growing and ripening of crops, summer to winter, life to death or incarnation to reincarnation, and is present in the coexistence of good and evil, male and female, sun and shade, wet and dry and hot and cold. As a part of this totality we are no less ordered by the *Tao* and subject to the interplay of *yin* and *yang* than any other part of the natural world. In nature an imbalance of *yin* and *yang* results in drought, storms, tidal waves, earthquakes and other disasters: in our own bodies it results in disease. Until we can grasp this essential relationship of man and cosmos we cannot begin to comprehend the basic concepts of Traditional Chinese Medicine or acupuncture.

Fundamental to the existence of all life on earth is water. Its movement can be traced from the smallest spring or well to tiny brooks which become streams and cascade into lakes, which give rise to slow majestic rivers, which wind their way to find the open sea. From the ocean, the water evaporates and forms vapour or mist which later becomes cloud. Finally, by the action of the wind and changes in temperature, the cloud condenses and falls as rain or snow upon the earth to be absorbed and, eventually, to complete the cycle. The Chinese realised that our own vital force or *qi*, as they called it, followed somewhat similar phases within the body (see Table 6 in chapter 3). These concepts of cyclical movement and change, the reflection of the universe and man in each other, and the interaction between them, are seminal to the whole of Traditional Chinese Medicine. Moreover, they provide the key to the recognition and understanding of the patterns of disease or disharmony as well as to the formulation of treatment. However, acupuncture can be practised in ignorance or defiance of traditional thinking: a topic which will be explored in greater depth later in this book.

THE ACUPUNCTURE RENAISSANCE
Since 1949, information about acupuncture has been finding its way into the

Western world with increasing vigour. In 1959, one of the first serious treatises on the subject appeared in the English language and, in 1960, a group of osteopaths and naturopaths who had studied acupuncture in France and Germany brought the famous Dr Lavier from France, and a number of practitioners attended his course on acupuncture in the UK. An Acupuncture Research Association was founded and, later, the Acupuncture Association, now the British Acupuncture Association, was inaugurated. In 1964 the Acupuncture Association set up its first college where doctors and osteopaths and others of similar medical standing could take a postgraduate course in acupuncture. Five years later the Acupuncture Research Association and the Acupuncture Association combined and opened a new college in London which is now the British College of Acupuncture. More recently, other colleges have been opened and several medical groups run courses for doctors, most of which are of very short duration. One of the earliest books on acupuncture in the English language was written by Felix Mann, who has now had five books on the subject published. Two other early authors of books on acupuncture were Mary Austin and Denis Lawson-Wood, both of whom are members of the British Acupuncture Association. In the last few years numerous books on acupuncture have been written and published, including several very scholarly works by Royston Low, the Dean of the British College of Acupuncture, and others by Jeremy Ross, Roger Newman Turner, Sidney Rose-Neil and Walter Thompson, who are members of the Association.

One of the recent political developments in British Acupuncture has been the establishment of a joint 'Register of British Acupuncturists' which lists well over five hundred qualified acupuncturists in Britain.

Developments in acupuncture in other countries are detailed in the Appendix.

2   *Outline of Acupuncture Philosophy*

As mentioned in chapter one, many of the early ideas basic to Chinese Medicine are enshrined in the *Nei Jing*, in which the accumulated wisdom found in miscellaneous writings were attributed in retrospect to the legendary Emperor Huang Ti and set out in the form of a dialogue between himself and his Chief Minister, Ch'i Po. The most important of these concepts were the *Tao, yin* and *yang*, the five elements or transformations and the eight principles or patterns of disharmony.

THE *TAO* AND THE 'WAY' TO WELL-BEING

The *Tao*, which, in Chinese, means the 'way', is seen as the motive force which calls forth order from primeval chaos. By the activity of the two polar forces of *yin* and *yang* creation is accomplished. After creation the Tao remains as the abstract, inconceivable influence which continues to exercise government over the universe, whilst *yin* and *yang*, through their dynamic interplay, maintain all things in their correct and harmonious balance.

The *Tao* contrasts with the Judao-Christian God in not being distinct from creation and not possessing the attributes of 'father' which lead to a possible response to prayer or intercession.

DISHARMONY AND DISEASE

Wrong-doing is not seen in the moralistic sense of Judaism, Christianity or Islam, in which punishment will eventually be meted out by an offended God, but is seen as something that insults creation by introducing disharmony. It therefore brings unhappiness and disease and prevents the individual from achieving the right goal or attaining perfection. The man who robs a bank, for example, because he is motivated by greed can never be happy and, for all his material gain, is nevertheless in a poorer state than the peasant who is contented in his mind and happy. The man who ignores the laws of nature and overeats, over-indulges in sex, takes no exercise, drinks excessive amounts of alcohol or takes other drugs, brings disharmony to his body directly as well as through his mind which lacks attunement to the universe and is consequently at variance with the *Tao*.

THE BASIS OF MODERN MEDICINE

In Chinese Traditional Medicine it is the dualistic principle of perfect harmony between *yin* and *yang* that is a fundamental and necessary part of creation, of being and of ideal health. It stands in stark contrast to the now rather outworn mechanistic model of Descartes and Newton which is the basis of modern science and modern scientific medicine. Whilst both have contributed much that is of value to mankind, the analytic process has failed to provide anything other than a purely superficial explanation of the universe and has dragged us into a cul-de-sac which has brought us to the verge of spiritual bankruptcy. It has regarded man as a machine, enabling him to be repaired when things go wrong; yet it has led him to be totally oblivious to the real cause of his problems and to disregard any attempt to search beyond the limits of physico-chemicalism to find the answer. It has, consequently, perpetrated ill-health simply because it has restricted man's understanding of himself, which has made him incapable of recognising the roots of his own disease. He has, therefore, been powerless to rectify the cause of his problems.

Orthodox medicine can be seen as concentrating on relatively unimportant matters and failing to get to the root of problems. As long ago as the 1920s, a certain Dr Fraser, The Canada Lancet 1926(?), demonstrated that bacteria were more likely to be the *result* of disease rather than its cause, but sixty years later we were still floundering with the discredited germ theory of Pasteur. Overwhelming evidence has been produced to show, for example, that undernutrition, malnutrition and environmental toxins are much more basic causes of 'infectious' diseases; yet destructive antibiotics are still being employed with an abandon which is beyond belief. It has been proved that acupuncture is capable of potentiating the immune response and enhancing resistance to so-called infections; yet nowhere in the Western world is it used to help people afflicted by such an illness.

TAOIST MEDITATION

A detailed account of Taoist meditation is far beyond the scope of this book; yet because of its importance within the totality of the Chinese medical system as well as a tool to promote understanding and well-being, a brief account of it is now included. Taoist meditation stems from the time of the legendary Huang Ti, the founder of Taoism, at a time when the mists of pre-history were hardly beginning to clear. However, the meditation which was revived by the philosopher Lao Tsu is central to Chinese medicine as it is directed to both the improvement of physical functioning and the attainment of greater enlightenment.

THE TECHNIQUE

Meditation should be done in a comfortable position with the spine erect and in an atmosphere of fresh air. The lotus or half lotus postures are recommended but for those for whom this is impossible there are good alternatives. The hands are crossed and rested gently on the lower legs with the thumb of the lower hand lightly grasping the palm of the upper hand. The chest should be slightly inclined forward and the buttocks pushed slightly backwards. The mouth remains closed and the tongue should just touch the roof of the mouth to conduct *prana* (energy from the air) from the nostrils to the throat. Eyes should be lightly closed or semi-closed. The mind is now cleared of all thoughts and desires and is brought to concentrate on nothing. Thoughts should not be actively forced out of the mind, for this is a sure way of causing them to return, but gently discouraged until they disappear. This type of meditation is an exercise in concentration but is also a method of cultivating the free movement of energy within the body. The *prana* which was mentioned earlier is another oriental term which refers to the subtle energy extracted from the air which ultimately goes to form the *qi*, the harmonious distribution of which is synonymous with good health.

MERIDIAN MEDITATION

The Chinese also described Meridian Meditation which consists of visualising and concentrating upon the meridians or pathways of energy which traverse the body. Sometimes this is assisted by physically rubbing or massaging the meridians with the thumbs following the traditional route from the meridian associated with the lungs where the flow of energy is said to commence, via each meridian in its rightful sequence (see Figure 6) ending with the liver meridian. The tips of the fingers may be used instead of the thumb and each side of the body should be done separately. Usually, the massage is performed first, after which one mentally travels through each meridian, sensing any blockage or disturbance of energy.

The meditation was part of what was known as the Internal Exercises which also included the three Animal Exercises taken from the deer, crane and turtle, all of which were observed to possess longevity. These exercises formed the basis of the Internal Exercises.

The Deer Exercise is based upon tightening and strengthening the anal muscles, which in the male strengthens the rectum and prostate, ameliorates impotence and premature ejaculation and helps to enlarge the head of the penis, and in the female strengthens the muscles of the vagina and rectum, cures and prevents many vaginal problems and menstrual disorders and helps to maintain youthfulness and beauty by strengthening the sexual glands. In both sexes the entire glandular system is energised and balanced by this exercise.

The Crane Exercise is essentially an abdominal breathing exercise and may be combined with the Deer Exercise. It is particularly helpful in calming the body and is a useful preparation for sleep.

The Turtle Exercise consists basically of stretching the neck in imitation of the tortoise pulling its head out of its shell. It energises the spine, including the neck, strengthens the shoulders and removes stiffness from the muscles in these areas. It also stimulates and regulates the thyroid and parathyroids: the very important endocrine glands sited in the neck region.

YIN AND *YANG* AND HEALTH

In Chinese philosophy it was thought that under the influence of *Tao* the original state of chaos became organised and energy was divided into two forces, *yin* and *yang*, which resulted in the formation of the material world. These two polar forces maintain everything in its rightful state by their continual ebb and flow, opposition and attraction and dynamic interplay. The entire cosmos became divided into heaven (*yang*) which consists of the light, ephemeral, 'pure' substance which rose upwards; and earth (*yin*) consisting of the heavier, coarser material which sank below. Thus, *yang* equates to the qualities of activity and function; whereas *yin* equates to those of passivity and structure. In one sense *yang* is life and *yin* is death, but even in death there is some *yang*, and in traditional Chinese thinking all things have life. There can be no *yin* without *yang* nor *yang* without *yin!*

The original explanation of *yin* was 'the shady side of a hill' or the north side (at least in the northern hemisphere) and *yang* was the sunny side or south. Thus, *yin* refers to dark, cold and damp; whilst *yang* refers to light, warm and dry. To take this a little further, *yin* stands for night and *yang* for day. The outer circle in Figure 1 depicts this relationship, whilst the intermediate circle depicts the relationship of yin and yang as determined by the cycle of the sun. From the moment of its descent from its zenith (moment of maximum *yang*) the *yin* force begins to increase. Conversely,

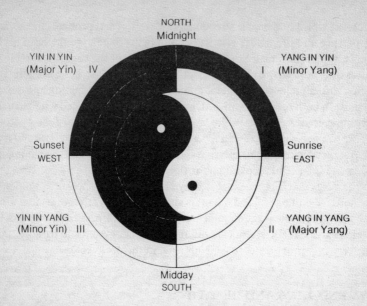

Figure 1 A schematic representation of the endless interplay of yin *and* yang. *The outer circle represents the daily variation of* yin *and* yang, *the intermediate circle portrays the solar cycle from zenith to nadir, and the inner circle is the Chinese monad showing how all things are composed of* yin *and* yang, *that* yin *changes into* yang *and vice versa, and that there is no* yin *without* yang *or* yang *without* yin.

TABLE 1
General and cosmological correspondences to yin *and* yang.

YIN	YANG
Earth	Heaven
Moon (Major *Yin*)	Sun (Major *Yang*)
Night	Day
Autumn/Winter	Spring/Summer
North	South
Noon-MN	MN-Noon
Completion	Incipience
Structure	Function
Passive	Active
Dark	Light
Wet	Dry
Cold	Hot
Proton	Electron
Negative	Positive
Sinking	Rising

20

TABLE 2
Some physiological features in terms of yin *and* yang.

YIN	YANG
Female	Male
Right side	Left side
Front	Back
Lower part	Upper part
Inside	Outside
Responsive	Aggressive
Transporting organs	Storage organs
Chronic	Acute
Deep pain	Superficial pain
Constant pain	Intermittent pain
Pain does not move	Pain moves around
Parasympathetic	Sympathetic
Centripetal	Centrifugal

from midnight, which is the moment of maximum *yin*, the *yang* influence begins to strengthen.

Everything in the universe can be perceived in terms of *yin* and *yang*. Table 1 lists some of the *yin/yang* correspondences in nature, whilst Table 2 shows how various anatomical and physiological characteristics may be understood in terms of *yin* and *yang*. The importance of this in respect of treatment should already be apparent.

PHYSIOLOGICAL CONSIDERATIONS

An intermittent (*yang*) pain which changes position, is superficial, aggravated by pressure and probably associated with inflammation is quite different from a constant, deep (*yin*) pain which does not move from place to place, is usually relieved by pressure and probably associated with degeneration. The treatment of such pains would also be different and, on the simplest level, the first type of pain would probably be relieved by a cold application and the second type with a hot one. However, nothing in medicine, Chinese or otherwise, should be taken for granted!

Table 3 lists a number of more objective anatomical and physiological correspondences, all of which help the physician to make a correct diagnosis in terms of Traditional Chinese Medicine.

Returning to Figure 1, we can observe that the daily cycles of sunrise and sunset initiate the qualities of major *yang*, minor *yang*, major *yin* and minor

TABLE 3

Yin *and* Yang *physiological manifestations. In general,* yang *manifestations are signs of good health, but excessively* yang *characteristics are also undesirable.*

PART OF BODY	YIN	YANG
Hair	White/Grey	Red/black
Head	Bald	Abundant hair
Eyes	Large, round	Long, thin
	Glazed	Sparkling
Eyebrows	Thin	Thick
Nose	Long	Short
Ears	Small	Large
	Small lobes	Large lobes
Lips	Thin or swollen	Thick (not swollen)
	Dark colour	Pink colour
Tongue	Flat	Roundish
	Quivering	Firm
	Protrudes little	Protrudes well
Joints	Stiff	Flexible
Hands	Hot/moist	Dry
	Cold & moist	Warm & dry
Nails	Long & narrow	Short & wide
	Grain across	Grain up & down
Skin	Smooth	Rough

yin. These variations of *yin* and *yang* are also important and are correlated to the organs and meridians.

Above all, it is the balance of these two contrasting forces which is important and it is this balance that changes according to the time of day, season of the year, age and sex of the individual and, even, the movement of the moon, planets and stars.

YIN AND *YANG* ORGANS

It was noted earlier that *yang* and *yin* were described as the sunny and shady sides of a hill. In place of the hill we can consider a man standing with his back to the sun. The back is then relatively *yang* and the front relatively *yin*. Since the small intestine and bladder meridians pass over the back (including the back of the arms and legs) these are regarded as great *yang*. Situated at the side are the 'three heater' and gall bladder meridians – these are considered as lesser *yang*. In the front, where the sun scarcely touches but its warmth is still felt, are the colon and stomach. These are sunlight *yang*. In the front of the body are lung and spleen; as they are in the most *yin* position they are

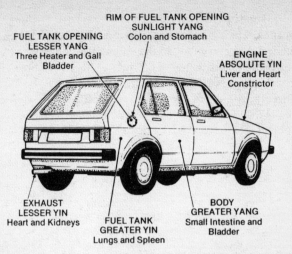

RIM OF FUEL TANK OPENING
SUNLIGHT YANG
Colon and Stomach

FUEL TANK OPENING
LESSER YANG
Three Heater and Gall
Bladder

ENGINE
ABSOLUTE YIN
Liver and Heart
Constrictor

EXHAUST
LESSER YIN
Heart and Kidneys

FUEL TANK
GREATER YIN
Lungs and Spleen

BODY
GREATER YANG
Small Intestine and
Bladder

Figure 2   Quality of yin *and* yang *in different areas shown by analogy with a car.*

termed great *yin*. A little more to the side are the heart constrictor and liver meridians which are absolute *yin*, whilst the heart and kidney are seen as lesser *yin* as they tend to be more posterior.

We can take a motor car to construct an analogy (see Figure 2). The outside is bathed in sunlight and is great *yang*. The rim of the petrol tank inlet is lesser *yang*, whilst the petrol cap is sunlight *yang*. As we descend into the petrol tank we pass through great *yin*. The engine is absolute *yin* and the exhaust, which is in contact with the outside, is lesser *yin*. According to Chinese medicine the lesser *yin* organs had to be deep in the body and contain rapidly flowing substance. Moreover, they had to be in contact with the outside. The two organs which fit these requirements are the heart and kidney. Absolute *yin* is the linking area between lesser *yin* and great *yin*. Since the great *yin* is the foundation of everything hidden and mysterious, the lungs and spleen were considered as great *yin*, and the liver and heart constrictor as absolute *yin*, which connects lesser *yin* and great *yin*. The liver lies between the pancreas (which is incorporated in the Chinese concept of spleen) and the right kidney, whilst the heart constrictor or pericardium undoubtedly lies snugly between the heart and lungs. The absolute *yin* is the foundation of greatness and honesty. In Western thought the heart figures in both these qualities but the liver tends to be ignored.

With respect to the *yang* organs, the stomach and colon are sunlight *yang*,

23

which is the foundation of everything and permeates everything. Digestion and elimination, which is begun by the stomach and completed by the colon, is the foundation of everything in the economy of the physical body. The lesser *yang* is the foundation of and brings to life the orifices of *yin*. The 'three heater' and gall bladder are regarded as lesser *yang* because they are situated deeply within the *yin* regions of the body and are, as it were, expressions of the *yin* activity. Great *yang* is the foundation of existence from the beginning to the end and comprises the bladder and small intestine.

TABLE 4

Classification of foods according to their relative yin *and* yang *qualities.*

YIN	YANG
Fruits	Grains
Leafy vegetable	Root vegetable
Sugar	Salt
Fluids/juices	Herb teas
Tea/coffee	Nuts & seeds
Alcohol	Meat/fish/cheese
Drugs/'chemicals'	Eggs
Raw food	Cooked food
Yoghurt	Miso
Spicy foods	Bitter foods

The food we eat (see Table 4) may also be analysed in terms of *yin* and *yang* instead of the more conventional, analytical method, and it can be seen that diet will also play an important part in harmonising the *yin* and *yang*. An entire 'science' of nutrition termed macrobiotics has grown up around this concept and, although the author does not agree with all the ideas expressed by exponents of this type of diet, many of the basic ideas are undoubtedly very valuable. Eating foods which are either extremely *yin* or extremely *yang*, such as sugar or salt, are likely to bring about imbalances: a belief shared by all naturopaths and now fully vindicated by science. A corollary to this theory that only locally grown food should be consumed seems to have a commonsense basis, but the application of it in our modern world is too difficult and inhibiting for most people. It may reasonably be questioned whether a rigid adherence to such a philosophy pays off. The axiom 'moderation in all things' might perhaps apply here and it can be argued that if predominantly locally grown produce is consumed, limited excursions into foods from different areas and other countries will do no harm.

3   *The Laws of Acupuncture and the Basis of Treatment*

THE LAW OF THE FIVE ELEMENTS

According to traditional Chinese thinking, when creation took place the *yin* and the *yang* brought forth the five elements of water, wood, fire, earth and metal which made up the material substance of everything in the world. The interaction of *yin* and *yang*, balanced by the *Tao*, ensured that the proportion of these elements was correctly maintained. Even though the concept of the five elements is a medieval one, this idea of how the universe is constructed has not only stood the test of time but is a source of great insight and understanding to those who take the trouble to study it. We shall now briefly examine some of the special meanings of the elements in acupuncture diagnosis and treatment.

WATER

Water is basic to life on this planet. In man it is the fluids of the body which nourish and maintain the health of every cell and if these fluids become obstructed or toxic the result is disease, degeneration and, ultimately, death. It is not surprising that the kidney, which is said to store the ancestral energy, is especially linked to this element. Water is the most *yin* of all the elements and is the main component of man as it is the source of nourishment and maintains the body. The movement of water in a fountain evokes a form and, in a similar way, the element water gives form to the body. Water corresponds to the vital fluids, blood, lymph, mucus, semen and fat. Being the universal solvent it cleanses as well as nourishes. It is associated with the kidneys, which nourish the bones, with the special sense of hearing, and with head hair. It is adversely affected by cold and it manifests a dark colour of violet or black. It nourishes the wood and exercises a controlling action upon fire (*see* Figure 3). When in balance there will be healthy teeth and hair, good hearing and sexual vitality.

WOOD

This represents the vegetative life within man: all the activities that continue

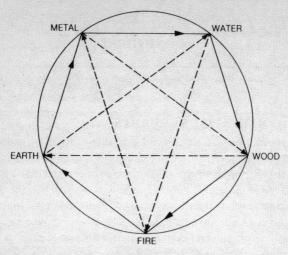

Figure 3   The five phases depicted as the five elements related by the sheng *or nutrition cycle (continuous line) and the* ko *or inhibiting cycle (dotted line).*

when unconscious such as digestion, heart beat, respiration and basic metabolism. In particular it relates to the activity of growing and increasing, and may be regarded as the 'spring' phase of life. When in balance it should give the strength of a tree combined with the suppleness of a sapling. It is associated with the liver which feeds the muscles, tendons and ligaments, and is related to the eyes. It nourishes fire and controls earth (by covering and penetrating it).

FIRE

Fire symbolises the combustion that takes place within the body, functions which have reached a stage of maximum activity and are about to decline, and also the higher spirit of psychic aspects of man. It is associated with the heart which nourishes the circulatory system and is related to the tongue or sense of speech. When in balance there will be equanimity of spirit, a sound mind and a healthy circulation. It nourishes earth (fire creates earth by producing ash) and controls metal (by melting it). It is adversely affected by excess heat.

EARTH

Earth is the symbol of stability or being properly anchored. Water, wood, fire and metal all have their relative positions in respect to earth. In the macrocosm without water there would be no visible life; without wood or vegetation the earth would be barren and human life could not be supported; without fire or warmth the world would be a frozen waste; and without metal the earth would be sterile. Earth is associated with the spleen which nourishes the connective tissue and is related to the sense of taste. When in balance the individual is mentally stable, contented, and experiences physical and social well-being. Earth nourishes metal (it gives rise to the metallic elements such as sodium, potassium, magnesium, iron, zinc, calcium and other essential nutrients) and controls water by damming and filtering it.

METAL

Symbolically, metal has a cutting and reforming action but it also refers to the solidifying process. In this aspect it can be seen as in opposition to fire and, clearly, the balance is again important. Metal elements are also donors of electrons and in this sense metal, although very *yin*, vivifies and produces *yang*. It nourishes water (it becomes liquid under the influence of fire, but it also dissolves in water) and controls wood (metal cuts wood). It is associated with the lungs which nourish the skin and are related to the nose and sense of smell. Those in whom metal is well balanced are strong, have healthy

TABLE 5
Some correspondences to the five elements.

ELEMENT	WOOD	FIRE	EARTH	METAL	WATER
VISCERA	Liver	Heart	Spleen	Lungs	Kidneys
ASSOCIATED ORGAN	Gall bladder	Small instestine	Stomach	Colon	Bladder
TISSUE	Muscle/ ligaments	Vascular system	Connective tissue	Skin	Bone/ teeth
ORIFICE	Eyes	Ears	Mouth	Nose	Genitalia/ anus
SENSE	Sight	Speech	Taste	Smell	Hearing
REFLECTED IN	Nails	Complexion	Lips	Body hair	Head hair
FLUID	Tears	Sweat	Lymph	Mucus	Saliva
ODOUR	Rancid	Burnt	Sweet	Fleshy	Putrid
EMOTION	Anger	Joy	Empathy	Grief	Fear
SEASON	Spring	Summer	Midsummer	Autumn	Winter
ADVERSE WEATHER	Wind	Heat	Humid/ damp	Dry	Cold
VOICE	Shouting	Laughing	Singing	Weeping	Groaning

skins, healthy assimilation and elimination and are resistant to disease.

INFLUENCE OF CLIMATE ON HEALTH

To the ancient Chinese climatic factors were the principal external disease-causing factors and, for this reason, much of their medical literature abounds with discussions about the weather! This is not as odd as it first sounds because a great deal of scientific investigation has now been carried out on the connection between disease and climate, season and weather, and some very interesting facts have emerged. The Mistral (wind) of the Mediterranean causes migraine, insomnia, recurrence of neuralgia, aggravation of tuberculosis and bronchitis. Hippocratic medicine speaks of pains which occur prior to changes in the weather and patients who can predict the weather by their own symptoms are well known. Surgeons know that complications to surgery occur more frequently at certain times and a study by Dr J. Kummel, in 1936, showed that operations are most dangerous when the weather is changing. It is well established that rheumatism is aggravated by sudden falls in temperature, strong winds and the influx of polar air masses, a discovery first made by Dr Tromp in the Netherlands. Asthma is vulnerable to the influence of the weather and is probably aggravated by an increase in the relative proportion of positive ions in the atmosphere and by lowering of the barometric pressure below a certain level. It is also sometimes aggravated by pollen which may account for its high incidence in the summer. Deaths from heart disease occur more often in very hot or very cold weather.

The Chinese believed that cold was particularly harmful to the functions and organs related to water and it is common experience that cold adversely affects the kidneys and bones – hence the expressions 'chill on the kidneys' and 'chilled to the bone'. The wood was thought to be particularly vulnerable to the East wind and the invasion of wind gives rise to aches and pains in the muscles and ligaments which tend to move around the body. Fire is aggravated by heat, earth by humidity and metal by dryness. Respiratory conditions are known to be made worse by very dry conditions and the skin is also not at its best when the weather is very dry.

THE FIVE ELEMENTS AND THE EMOTIONS

A healthy emotional state was recognised by the Chinese as being the indispensable condition of good general health and to them the correct balance of assertiveness, joy, calmness, sympathy, and respect were essential.

Excessive anger, excessive joy or excitement, obsession, prolonged or disproportionate grief and fearfulness or anxiety were the internal adverse factors which resulted in disease. More correctly, they are the manifestation of imbalances in the five elements caused by internal factors and represent a weakness or fixation in one of the elements.

Anger is related to wood and this is reflected in our use of the word 'liverish'. Inability to express anger is seen as a weakness in the wood.

Excessive joy or excitement is seen as harmful to the fire and the association between joy and fire must be more than mere imagination since the heart 'jumps for joy' and 'misses a beat' from excitement. Lack of joy or lack of *joie de vivre* is a depressive state related to the fire and can often be dramatically cured by a simple tonification of the heart meridian. The earth is related to the centre and 'being centred' or properly grounded allows us to experience empathy and calmness.

Inability to concentrate and the 'grasshopper' mind may be caused by problems with the stomach or spleen which are related to earth. In this connection, it cannot be emphasised too greatly or too often that the Chinese were not speaking of the precise anatomical organs as we understand them today, but to physiological functions connected more with the *qi* or vital energy (for a fuller explanation, see chapter 4) than the gross, visible material structure or corresponding physiology.

Grief, we know, affects the lungs. One gasps or holds one's breath on hearing bad news, whilst skin conditions are well known to be aggravated by anxiety. Prolonged or disproportionate grief is a recognisable type of depression and the focus of treatment in these cases must be the lungs.

Finally, it needs no prompting from me to remind the reader of the physiological effects of excessive fear. Even before giving a lecture a well-known and experienced professor confided in the author that he always had to visit the lavatory before a performance. The widespread occurrence of anxiety in modern times, especially in women, is great cause for alarm because it probably reflects the prevalent abuse of our health which may diminish the inherited 'ancestral *qi*' which is stored in the kidneys. It may, also, have something to do with the exorbitant quantities of salt consumed by people today because salt is the flavour related to this element. Similarly, the flavour of sweetness is associated with earth which encompasses the spleen-pancreas. It is evident that diabetes, a disease of the pancreas, is closely related to sugar intake which has experienced an astronomical rise over the last hundred years or so. During the war years in Europe, when sugar was

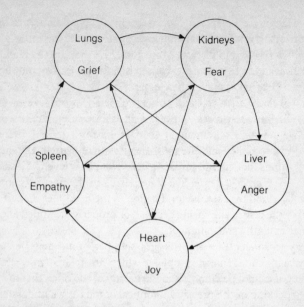

Figure 4   The relationship of the zang (yin) *organs in accordance with the* sheng *and* ko *cycles and the corresponding emotions.*

rationed, diabetes declined at the same rate with the consumption of sugar.

It is noteworthy that according to the *ko* cycle (shown in Figure 4), anger overcomes sympathy, joy overcomes grief, empathy or sympathy overcomes fear, grief overcomes anger and fear overcomes joy. How many people lead joyless lives because they are racked by anxiety or fear and how many criminals, thugs and delinquents are ill because of imbalances in their energy which could easily be put right by acupuncture and correct nutrition? Drugs, electroconvulsive therapy and prison have all been tried and found wanting but for some obscure reason no society has yet been brave enough to substitute these measures with economically sounder and more promising treatment outlined in Chinese medicine!

Some of the acupuncture points which are particularly helpful in regulating the energy on the basis of an appraisal of the five elements are mentioned in Table 6.

THE MOTHER-SON LAW

This is another idea concerning the five elements and the relationship

TABLE 6

Points relating to the five elements or phases on each of the principal meridians.

(1) DESCRIPTION CHINESE	(2) ENGLISH	(3) YANG	(4) YIN	(5) APPROX. LOCATION	(6) ENERGIC STATE	(7) MOST USEFUL FOR:
Jing	Well	Metal	Wood	Tips of fingers/ toes	Energy is at its most mutable point	Mental illness
Yong	Brook	Water	Fire	Hands/feet	Energy is more specifically polar	Febrile illness
Yu	Stream	Wood	Earth	Hands/feet	Energy flows more strongly	Painful joints
Ching	River	Fire	Metal	Wrist/ankle	Energy concentrates	Respiratory disorders
Ho	Sea	Earth	Water	Elbow/Knee	Energy emerges from or enters a deeper level	Digestive disorders

Column 1 lists the Chinese description, column 2 gives the approximate English equivalent, columns 3 and 4 tell the polarity of the meridian, column 5 notes the approximate anatomical position, column 6 shows the level or state of energy at that stage and column 7 indicates the most useful therapeutic indication. These points are most suitable for manipulating the energy and are frequently employed for treatment based upon a diagnosis of the relative state of the five phases.

between them. It would better be described as a working hypothesis rather than a law. In fact it is nothing more than the *sheng* cycle since it proposes that the liver is the 'mother' of the heart, the heart the 'mother' of the spleen, the spleen-pancreas the 'mother' of the lungs, the lungs the 'mother' of the kidneys and the kidneys the 'mother' of the liver. The same relationship exists between the gall bladder and small intestine, the stomach and colon, the bladder and gall bladder, which are the 'coupled' organs.

A problem manifested by any organ in the body is thought to be due to its not being properly nourished by the 'mother'. A lung disorder, for example, is seen as a failure of the heart to transmit vital energy or *qi* to the lungs: an explanation which is by no means inconsistent with Western medical thinking.

RHYTHM ROUND THE CLOCK

Every day consists of four intervals – morning, afternoon, evening and night. These daily divisions are like miniature seasons of spring, summer, autumn and winter. Thus, the annual rhythm of life is influenced by this daily variation. The significance of this is considerable and a great many scientific papers have been devoted to this topic. The weather is also influenced by this cycle: strong winds abate in the evening and storms are more frequent in the late afternoon. All our bodily functions vary according to the time of day. For example, blood levels of melatonin, a hormone secreted by the pineal gland, are high at night and low during the day. This, in turn, causes reduction in the activity of the ovaries at night. Blood pressure and body temperature are higher in the evening than they are in the early morning – at least in healthy people. Babies tend to be born in the early hours of the morning, and it has been established that it is actually easier to give birth at that time than at other periods of the day. It is interesting that more people die at this time as well!

According to Traditional Chinese Medicine, there is a surge of vital energy or *qi* in each organ in every two hour period of every twenty-four hour cycle. This starts in the lungs between 3-5 am because the expansion of the lungs signifies the drawing of energy into the system. Apparently, we should be born during those hours! There is little doubt that the time of birth is significant and should be under the control of the foetus. The postponement of birth to 'office' hours is thought by traditional practitioners and modern doctors alike to be disadvantageous to the baby.

Coinciding with the Chinese clock, symptoms of excess will be aggravated at the time of fullness of energy, whilst those of deficiency may be aggravated at the opposite period of the day when the organ energy is at its minimum. These periods are used to treat the relevant organs and there are even specific points on each of the twelve main meridians or channels where this may be best carried out. These are known as horary points. On each meridian, there are points which relate preferentially to each of the five elements or phases and the horary point is the one which relates to the element of that particular organ and for that reason is also known as the 'element' point. In a deficiency state the point is used at the beginning of the two hour period when the

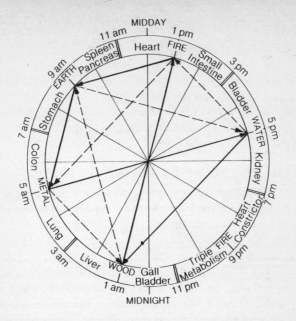

Figure 5 The Chinese Clock. This indicates the periods of optimal energy in the different phases and related organs or functions. Superimposed upon this are the sheng *(nutrition) cycle, denoted by the continuous heavy line and the* ko *(inhibitory) cycle, denoted by the intermittent line. The faint lines traversing the centre denote the Midday Midnight Relationship.*

energy is starting its surge. In excess conditions the point is treated with a sedating technique at the end of the period.

THE MIDDAY-MIDNIGHT LAW

It would be inconvenient to treat the liver during its appropriate period, which is in the early hours of the morning, and even the most dedicated doctor would not take kindly to his patients turning up at 3 am to have their lungs toned up. As a rule, patients do not turn up for treatment during the hours of night which is an extremely good thing. Fortunately, according to the Midday-Midnight Law a patient who has liver problems and requires treatment between 1 am and 3 am can come and have exactly the opposite treatment done to his small intestine at the same hours in the afternoon. The Chinese doctors obviously realised that without such a law they would get no sleep, and even if it had not been discovered it would surely have had to have

33

been invented. Figure 5 shows the Chinese clock and the implications of the Midday-Midnight Law can easily be seen from this.

It is of great academic interest that when the *sheng* and *ko* cycle relationships are placed into this picture, these both form numerous regular geometric patterns, a phenomenon which, to the best of the author's knowledge, has not previously been noted. It contributes nothing to any medical or therapeutic application of these laws but enhances a little the theory that God is a mathematician.

THE HUSBAND-AND-WIFE LAW

According to Traditional Chinese Medicine, half the organs of the body are reflected in the pulse at the left wrist and the other half at the right wrist. There are three positions and at least two levels at each pulse. The three positions are approximately one finger's width apart. The levels are superficial and deep. The superficial level can be felt by very lightly touching the skin. The deep level can be felt by pressing hard enough almost to obliterate the pulse. Each level at each position reflects a different organ which is shown in Table 7. The organs associated with the pulses on the left side are designated 'husband'; whilst those associated with the right side are 'wife'. (Remember, women are always in the *right*.) In health, the husband should be dominant and the wife submissive. The sexist terminology is used to explain an underlying truth about the relationships between the organs. If a 'wife' dominates a 'husband' the seed of disorder has already been sown.

The acupuncturist learns a great deal about the energy in the different organs from the pulses and that is why he will sometimes spend quite a lot of time feeling the different pulses. It doesn't mean, as some patients think, that he can't find the pulse!

TABLE 7
The left and right pulses showing the related organs and the Husband-and-Wife Law.

POSITION	LEVEL	'HUSBAND' LEFT WRIST	'WIFE' RIGHT WRIST
Distal	Deep	Heart	Lungs
	Superficial	Small intestines	Colon
Medial	Deep	Liver	Spleen-pancreas
	Superficial	Gall bladder	Stomach
Proximal	Deep	Kidneys	Heart constrictor
	Superficial	Bladder	Triple metabolism

4   Qi, *Organs, Meridians and Acupuncture Points*

WHAT IS *QI*?

It has already been mentioned that the term *qi* or *ch'i* is the name given by the Chinese to denote the subtle energic principle which activates the body and maintains it in good health.

It is often very difficult for those of us who have been born and brought up in a modern Western society to appreciate the concept of *qi* when all our bodily functions are described in the analytical terms of physics and chemistry. The energy within the body is only understood as heat or electricity liberated from high energy molecules.

When the working of the body as a whole is considered, perhaps a good analogy is that of radio and television receivers which operate on two types of energy. On the one hand they both require electrical power either supplied by the mains or a battery; this source of power could be compared to the normal food of the human being. It is interesting that neither radio nor television can work without a measured current which, incidentally, even produces heat as food does in the body. On the other hand, and much more important to their proper function, however, are the radio and television waves which are subtle electromagnetic waves permeating the environment and which are 'absorbed' by the radio and television, and transmuted into a recognisable audible or visual display. The very existence of such waves would have been strongly denied by scientists of earlier centuries because there was no technology to recognise them. In fact, of course, many of them would not have existed since there was no broadcasting, but diffuse energy within these wavelengths has always existed, even if it remained obscure until our modern invention of the radio and television. Many other electromagnetic energies of various wavelengths abound in our universe and we can categorise these under the broad description of cosmic radiation. These cosmic energies are selectively absorbed by the human being and transmuted for his or her own benefit.

Paracelsus said that, 'The mere looking at externals is a matter for clowns, but the intuition of internals is a secret which belongs to physicians.' David Tansley in his book on radionics begins, 'Since ancient times man has held the belief that his physical body is simply the externalization of more subtle vehicles of manifestation. References to these invisible bodies are to be found in a wide variety of texts originating in China, India, Egypt and ancient Greece. The Bible too refers frequently to the subtle anatomy of man, particularly in *The Revelation of St John*.' A little further on he writes about the etheric body having three basic functions: 'It acts as a receiver of energies, an assimilator of energies and as a transmitter of energies. If each of these functions is maintained in a state of balance, then the physical body reflects this interchange of energies as a state of good health.' This very succinctly summarises the Chinese concept of *qi* and even its derangement, thought by the Chinese to be brought about by internal and external devils (adverse emotions and harmful environmental factors) which closely parallels Tansley's analogy of boulders jutting up from the bed of a stream, hindering the passage of the water.

Qi is said to be extracted from the food after it has been properly digested. This is done by the spleen, but if the food is not fully digested the *qi* is not properly refined and gross 'impure' substance will be sent by the spleen to different parts of the body where it will cause pollution, congestion and disease. This is another way of stating the fact that poor digestion is the foundation of disease. If the digestion is good, the *qi* is transported by the spleen to the lungs where it combines with ancestral *qi* from the kidneys and *qi* from the air to form the true *qi* of the body. This *qi* is sent to all parts of the body and it permeates the entire organism, initiating and sustaining movement, protecting the body from adverse invasive factors from the outside, constituting a warp to hold everything in place, maintaining normal temperature and generating the vital substances such as blood, urine, sweat, tears and semen. According to its function *qi* is differentiated into the following:

ORGAN *qi*

The *qi* in each of the organs is the same but functions differently in different organs in much the same way as radio waves might produce classical music on one channel on the radio, a debate on another and jazz on a third. A closer examination of the organs and functions will be made when we come to deal with the *zang fu*.

MERIDIAN *qi*

This is the *qi* or energy that is transmitted via the meridian network and is responsible for sustaining the body and contributing towards its material development.

PROTECTIVE *qi*

The protective *qi* circulates between the skin and flesh and is responsible for protecting the body from adverse external influences. It controls the pores of the body, moistens the skin and is involved in the production of sweat and urine.

NUTRITIVE *qi*

This is the energy which contributes to the formation of the blood and moves inseparably with the blood within the vessels.

ANCESTRAL *qi* AND SOURCE *qi*

Ancestral *qi* is the motivating force behind the nutritive and protective *qi*. It concentrates within the chest and aids the rhythmic movements of respiration and heart beat. This is the *qi* that moves the blood. Source *qi* is of congenital origin and is stored in the kidneys and is said to be the root of the twelve primary meridians and the fount of life.

DISTURBANCES OF *qi*

Stagnant qi   This is when the orderly movement of *qi* is impaired. When this occurs in the limbs it manifests itself as aches and pains. When it is in the organs it shows up in different ways as shown in Table 8.

TABLE 8

Some symptoms of stagnant and deficient qi *in the five* zang *(yin organ-systems).*

ORGAN	STAGNANT QI	DEFICIENT QI
Liver	Distension of chest and abdomen, digestive and menstrual disorders	Irritability, timidity, fear, indecision, blurred vision
Heart	Stabbing pain in left shoulder, cold hands and feet, blueness of lips	Spontaneous sweating, lethargy, shortness of breath
Spleen	Retention of urine, fullness or distension of chest & abdomen	Lassitude, muscular weakness, loss of appetite, oedema, diarrhoea
Lungs	Cough, shortness of breath	Weak cough, asthma, weakness of voice, fatigue
Kidneys	Incontinence, oedema	Backache, reduced sexual drive, shortness of breath

Rebellious qi This implies that the *qi* is going in the wrong direction. For example the *qi* of the spleen should go upwards, and if it reverses there may ultimately be prolapse of the abdominal or pelvic organs. Another manifestation is diarrhoea. On the other hand the *qi* of the stomach should go downwards, and if this is rebellious there will be vomiting. Rebellious *qi* is a subcategory of stagnant *qi*.

Deficient qi This may affect the entire body with resulting tiredness and lethargy, or may be in a particular organ (*see* Table 8).

Collapsed qi This is a subcategory of deficient *qi* and is manifested by prolapses.

BLOOD

It is extremely difficult to identify the difference between the Chinese concept of blood and the blood which we know circulates in our blood vessels. In fact they are much the same thing, but the Chinese concept of blood envisages a fluid which is not entirely confined to the blood vessels but even flows in the meridians. Blood is formed by the action of *qi* upon the elements of nutrition, having been transported by the spleen to the lungs and heart. There is a close relationship between the blood and *qi* and it is the *qi* that moves the blood. If the blood is deficient the face will be pale and lustreless, and the skin may become dry. In the heart a deficiency produces a dull, pale complexion, insomnia, poor memory and palpitations. In other organs it will produce other symptoms. The blood may also be stagnated or congealed, a condition often characterised by sharp, stabbing pains. There may be swelling of organs where there is congealed blood.

BODY FLUID

Known as *jin ye*, the body fluids are secreted by the cells of the body and include tears, sweat, saliva, milk, genital secretions, intestinal secretions and, perhaps most important of all, the secretions of the endocrine glands or hormones.

THE ORGANS

Zang fu is the name for the organ system in Chinese Medicine. Most of them are equated to the corresponding anatomical organs known to Western science but the Chinese concepts are slightly different, much wider and embrace functions not normally attributable to the organs in Western science (*see* Table 9). In addition, there is the triple metabolism, which is sometimes known as *the three heater,* and also the pericardium, which is known as *heart*

TABLE 9

The zang-fu *organs, their functions, and designations as State Officials.*

ORGAN	OFFICIAL	FUNCTIONS
Liver	Military General	Seat of the soul. Controls metabolism, removes toxins, stores blood. Sends pure energy to gall bladder.
Gall Bladder	Decision Maker	Receives pure energy from liver. Stores and secretes bile. Overactivity results in rash decisions, underactivity in indecision.
Heart	Emperor	Seat of all powers of mind and soul. Rules blood and vessels. Stores the *shen* (spirit).
Small intestine	Chief Executive	Separates pure from impure. Transforms matter into pure energy and waste. If it is in disharmony the body lacks nourishment and there is stagnation of thought.
Heart constrictor	Ambassador of Joy and Happiness	Protects the heart. Together with the three heater moves blood and *qi* throughout the body and harmonises its activity.
Three heater	Minister of Central Heating and Waterways	Controls body temperature. Together with heart constrictor enables all the other *zang fu* to function. Waterways probably refers to the lymph system.
Stomach	Official of Rotting and Ripening	Receives, rots and ripens the food. Sends 'pure' part to the spleen and the 'turbid' part to small intestines.
Spleen	Minister of Transport and Distribution	Transports energy throughout the body. Sends energy from food to the lungs. Moves and transports water.
Kidneys	Minister of Health and Social Security	Stores ancestral energy *(jing)*. Rules birth, growth and maturation. Rules water.
Bladder	Provincial Governor	Receives and excretes urine. Complements kidney and lower three heater.
Colon	Minister of Drains	Removes wastes from the body. Instigates change. Disharmony of colon results in a rigid type of thinking.
Lungs	Administrators of Orderly Conduct	Control *qi*. Seat of the 'soul' which more or less refers to nervous system. They also rule water and the outside of the body.

constrictor or *circulation sex*. The three heater refers more or less to the three types of metabolism going on in the body; namely the interchange of gases in the lungs and tissues which takes place in the upper heater, the digestion and metabolism of food which takes place in the middle heater, and the metabolism of elimination and sexual function which is the lower heater. The three heater is also intimately connected with what we call the endocrine system in Western physiology. The heart constrictor, as its various names suggest, is a sort of protector of the heart as well as being concerned with circulation and sexual function.

THE MERIDIANS

Jing luo is the system of meridians or channels which traverse the body and act as transmitters of *qi*. The twelve 'regular' meridians which are associated directly with the twelve organs are known as the main meridians. There are also eight 'extra' meridians, so called because they are ancillary to the principal meridians, although two of these which traverse the midline of the body and have their own points are included with the other twelve main meridians. The remaining six extra meridians have transits which coincide with portions or segments of the main meridians and they lack any independent points. They are sometimes known as lesser meridians. However, another name for them is miraculous meridians.

Symptoms experienced by a patient are often seen to be on a particular meridian, so it is vital for the acupuncturist to have an intimate knowledge of the precise pathway of every meridian in order that he can make a correct interpretation of such symptoms. Pain at the back of the head or in the neck or shoulders may be associated with the gall bladder or its meridian which traverses those areas; whereas pain in the face or teeth might be related to the stomach or colon meridians.

The main meridians are connected by joining vessels known as *lo* or *luo* meridians. These connect the coupled organs such as the lungs and colon and they join each meridian to its successor in the general circuit of energy around the body as portrayed by the Chinese clock (*see* Figure 5). So, for example, the colon meridian which ends around the nasal area is joined to the stomach meridian which originates just under the eye.

In addition to these meridians, there are also subsidiary vessels known as tendino-muscular meridians and distinct or divergent meridians. These follow similar pathways to the major meridians.

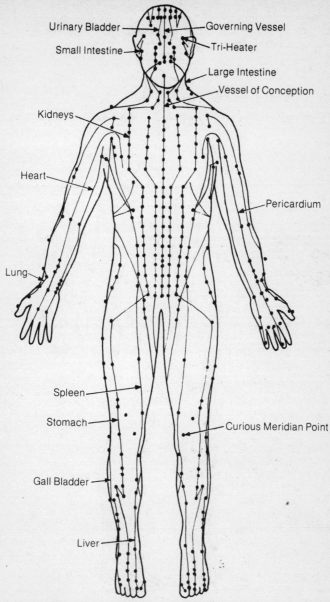

Urinary Bladder
Governing Vessel
Small Intestine
Tri-Heater
Large Intestine
Vessel of Conception
Kidneys
Heart
Pericardium
Lung
Spleen
Stomach
Curious Meridian Point
Gall Bladder
Liver

Figure 6   The meridians and acupuncture points. (Front view.)

41

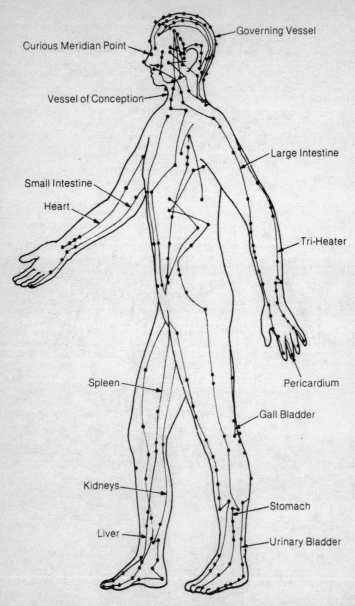

Curious Meridian Point

Governing Vessel

Vessel of Conception

Large Intestine

Small Intestine

Heart

Tri-Heater

Spleen

Pericardium

Gall Bladder

Kidneys

Stomach

Liver

Urinary Bladder

Figure 7   The meridians and acupuncture points. (Side view.)

42

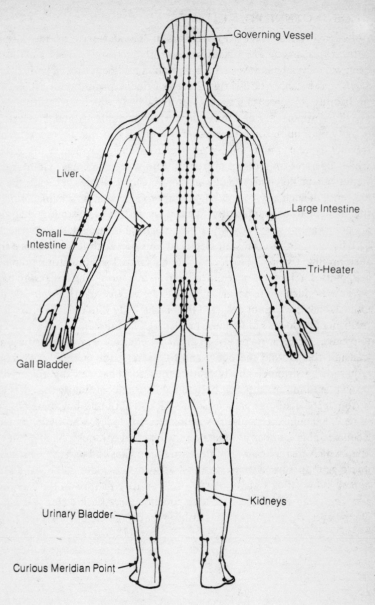

Figure 8   The meridians and acupuncture points. (Back view.)

43

ACUPUNCTURE POINTS

Although a Korean professor has claimed to have demonstrated the existence of the meridians and acupuncture points through tissue analysis, and this has been well developed by Walter Thompson in his book *Acupuncture as Far as We Know*, it cannot be asserted that this evidence is unquestionable. In all probability there are such routes within the body which are identifiable by peculiar proportions of DNA (deoxyribonucleic acid) and bioelectrical activity, and quite some time ago it was suggested that there was a 'data transfer system' much more primitive than the known nervous system, which operates on a direct current of miniscule amperage. Dr Margaret Patterson, in her book *Addictions can be Cured,* argues the case for the existence of such a system in her attempt to give a rational explanation for the phenomena of acupuncture. We can say with virtual certainty that there are points around the body which are recognisable through their bioelectric activity or ability to transmit electrical impulses with less resistance than surrounding tissue. The points can be termed acupuncture points or acupoints. Dr Thompson refers to them as 'acupores' which seems to me to be a very much more meaningful and descriptive name. After all, it is unlikely that the Creator designed the human body with points all over it for the benefit of doctors of Chinese medicine! The function of the acupores is to receive electromagnetic energy from the environment, to transmute and transmit this around the body, and to 'excrete' the energy which is not required. This would entirely validate the traditional view that the needles, when placed in the acupores, help to regulate and harmonise the energy.

About 365 acupores or points date back to antiquity but there are now some 2,000 points recognised by acupuncturists today. This figure includes a considerable number of points on the external ear, nose, hands, feet and scalp which are replications of the entire meridians and organs portrayed as micro acupuncture systems on small areas of the body: notably the sense organs. This reflex system may be used for acupuncture on the ears, nose and scalp, whilst on the feet the most common therapeutic action is massage. On the eyes, the phenomenon is utilised for diagnostic purposes only.

5 *Disease: Cause and Diagnosis*

CAUSES OF DISEASE

In terms of conventional medical thinking we can identify eight different factors which cause disease:

1   Genetic. (This compares with (9) below.)
2   Nutritional. This may be under-nutrition or malnutrition.
3   Metabolic. This includes tumours.
4   Infection.
5   Environmental. Includes exposure to environmental toxins and adverse climatic factors.
6   Structural. Trauma could be included under this heading.
7   Allergy. This could be regarded as a sub-category of metabolic disorder.
8   Wearing out.

In Chinese medical thinking the causes of disease are in many ways similar:

1   The external evil influences of wind, heat, fire, damp, dryness, and cold. (Similar to (5) above.)
2   The mental pathogens (internal devils) of anger, worry, anxiety, excessive grief, excessive fear and fright.
3   Epidemics. (Similar to (4) above.)
4   Bad foods and beverages. (Similar to (2) above.)
5   Excessive sexual activity.
6   Trauma from incidents such as animal bites and accidents. (Similar to (6) above.)
7   Visceral parasites.
8   Poisoning.
9   Hereditary factors.

The effect of adverse weather and emotions has already been discussed in chapter 3. Before the discovery of microorganisms in the West, the Chinese had a remarkable understanding of epidemics and realised that they could be spread by lack of ventilation, overcrowding, infected people or animals and contaminated water. The custom of drinking a lot of boiled water in the form of weak tea had its origins in this knowledge. Long before inoculation of smallpox was known in the West, the Chinese were using this form of immunisation against smallpox. The value of inoculation and vaccination is now uncertain, but it indicates that the Chinese displayed a considerable insight into the transmission of infections.

POOR NUTRITION

The question of nutrition has also already been mentioned in chapter 2 and there is no doubt at all that absolute priority should be given to the provision of adequate food and clean water for all populations. This is independent of acupuncture or any other therapy. Eating wisely is an integral precept of Chinese medicine which, as expected, stresses the importance of balance. It has already been noted how excessive salt and sugar consumption can harm people. In addition to that, the modern practices of refining, adding non-nutritive chemicals, overcooking, incorrect cooking, bad preparation, freezing, storing, preserving and mixing foods are all contributing daily to our ill-health. The poor nutritional quality of the food, together with other prevalent modern influences, encourages overeating – another serious and ubiquitous present-day nutritional source of disease. According to traditional medicine, food which is not properly digested in the stomach gives rise to contamination of the 'essence' or energy sent to the spleen and liver. This results in the body having to recruit exceptional methods of eliminating waste matter such as boils, skin eruptions, perspiration, etc. The condition may reach the stage where a fever is induced to 'burn up' this accumulated matter which often takes on the form of excess phlegm. The first, and best medicine is, therefore diet: either a restricted diet or a fast.

STRAIN

Another cause of disease is strain. According to the Chinese, too much walking strains the liver and gall bladder, which will be reflected in aching of the muscles and ligaments; too much looking affects the heart and small intestines and causes problems in the circulation; too much sitting injures the spleen and stomach which is noticed as sensitive flesh; too much lying down is detrimental to the lungs and colon, causing reactions on the skin; and too much standing injures the kidneys and bladder which results in aching bones.

The ancient thinkers were more or less unanimous in their condemnation of excessive sexual activity, and some of their modern equivalents go as far as to say that all sexual activity if brought to the point of normal orgasm is injurious to the health as it 'saps vital energy'. Others are obsessed with the harmful effects of masturbation, though, logically, it cannot be seen that this can have any different physical effect to 'normal' sexual intercourse. It cannot be agreed as to what constitutes excess with regard to this activity but there seems little doubt that over-indulgence in sex, just as in anything else, will bring about eventual ill-health. On the other hand, sex without orgasm is often recommended as enhancing health and various techniques and postures are prescribed for different problems.

THE BASIS OF ALL DISEASE

The root cause of all disease in terms of acupuncture is a disorder of vibration. Every cell in the body vibrates at a specific rate and vibration is, of course, energy. Vibrations outside the normal range are synonymous with disease. The insertion of needles aids the restoration of correct and harmonious vibration and in this way restores health.

HOW THE ACUPUNCTURIST MAKES A DIAGNOSIS

If you decide to visit an acupuncturist, what can you expect of him or her? After, I hope, making you welcome, he will listen very carefully to your history as any doctor should do. The only difference is that in addition to the usual questions asked by doctors about bowels, waterworks, appetite, sleeping habits, etc., he will ask what might seem to be some rather strange questions. No, he will not enquire about your heart constrictor or if you have a pain in your three heater, but he will want to know at what times your symptoms are worse, or for that matter better.

If you wake up every morning with discomfort at about 1.30 he will suspect that you have a nattering gall bladder because, according to the Chinese clock, that is the time when the gall bladder is likely to be most vocal. He will be particularly anxious to know if you are affected in any way by the weather; especially heat, cold, damp or the wind. If you dislike the cold, or fear the cold, or your symptoms are worse in cold weather, the acupuncturist will turn his attention to the kidneys and bladder which are more vulnerable to cold than any other organs.

Of course, he will not forget to ask you about your emotional state. If you tell him that you 'fly off the handle' easily he will suspect the liver or gall bladder; if you cry a lot he will probably think of the lungs, and if you are sad or anxious he will most likely be led to consider the spleen. He might want to know if you are attracted or repelled by any particular colour or taste because any positive reply to these questions would also be helpful in terms of assisting him to recognise a fixation in one of the elements.

The acupuncturist will take into consideration any medical tests which you have undergone. Some of these tests are of virtually no value but many of them are extremely useful. It cannot be stressed too often that acupuncture is not opposed to other forms of medicine, and especially not to modern medical investigations. This is why it is necessary for acupuncturists to have medical knowledge. A case to illustrate this occurred in Sri Lanka when an Oriental lady working in a developed country was being tutored on an advanced course of acupuncture. She carried out an acupuncture treatment on a man with a serious heart condition in which she stimulated the kidneys. Now we have already learned in chapter 3 that this will have a dampening effect upon the heart (water being put on the fire) and in this particular case it was obviously the wrong treatment. Had this lady been able to understand an electrocardiograph or taken the trouble to ask one of the many doctors who could, the treatment could have been modified accordingly. As it was, because of her ignorance and cynicism concerning Western medicine the man received a dangerous treatment. When subsequently questioned about this in her examination, the practitioner was rash enough to reply that the patient was fine after her treatment. What she did not know was that he was later taken into a coronary care unit.

Some of the author's colleagues maintain that acupuncture (provided it is carried out by a trained acupuncturist) cannot do any harm. This is because the acupuncture cannot induce the body to do anything detrimental to itself. In other words, the needles can only encourage the body towards a balance or harmonisation. The author would agree with this principle: the problem in the case just related is that the kidneys of that particular patient *did* need stimulating but the important factor was the correct order or priority of treatment. It is the author's belief that the order of priority can be changed by acupuncture or even by massage or touch for that matter. In this case we are imposing upon the body a new order of correction or, put more accurately, we are directing the body's healing force to deal with compensations rather than the prime problem. Normally this does not matter too much and the very worst that happens is that the patient takes longer to recover, but occasionally it can be disastrous.

To return to our visit to the acupuncturist, he will also ask you about perspiration, belching, wind, sexual habits and work. Having given all the answers you will then be asked to disrobe for an examination.

Once again, the examination will follow usual procedures with a number of additions. These are centred mostly on the tongue, the eyes, the pulses and specific reactive points called the alarm points. He will ask you to put out your tongue and will note whether it comes out with a good thrust or goes slowly with reluctance. The first type of movement is *yang* and is a good sign. The second is *yin* and not so good. He will note if the tongue goes out a good way or not very far. The same two considerations apply. Then he will look at the colour and shape of the tongue itself. It should be a nice pink colour and slightly rounded. A very flat tongue indicates a *yin* condition. Teeth marks, cracks, or scalloping around the edges are all significant and are signs that something is not quite right. If the colour is a bright pink or red it probably indicates an excessive *yang* condition; whereas if it is a purple colour there is stagnation and probably congealed blood. Table 10 lists some of the types of tongues and moss (covering) with their respective indications. The moss should be a delicate white colour – anything else is a sign of imbalance.

TABLE 10
A few simple tongue appearances with some corresponding disorders.

DESCRIPTION OF TONGUE	CONDITIONS
Bright red tongue	Symptoms due to heat:
Pale red tongue	Collapse of energy and blood which is often due to actual loss of blood
Purple tongue	Stagnation of *qi* and blood or excess blood
Pale tongue	Indication of *yin* condition. May be anaemia or malnutrition
Cleft tongue	Deficiency of blood, *qi* or true *yin*
Tooth marks on side (scalloping)	*Yang* deficiency or deficient *qi* of spleen and stomach
Fat tongue	Deficiency or cold
Quivering tongue	Injury to nervous system
Inability of tongue to protrude	Extreme weakness
Cracked tongue	Invasion of pathogenic heat

The moss (coating) may be white, yellow, grey or even black and the moss may be thick, thin, greasy or dry. Anything other than a thin white moss is abnormal.

The acupuncturist will now possibly look closely in your eyes. He is looking for signs in the iris which might give him a further clue to the basic problem causing your disorder. He might also carry out a normal opthalmoscopy in which he would look at the retina. He will then feel your pulses, a matter that has already been discussed in chapter 3. The ancient Chinese doctors would spend up to half an hour feeling these pulses and preferred to do it only at the crack of dawn, which are additional reasons for our placing less reliance on this nowadays.

The acupuncturist may now feel your abdomen. He might do a normal abdominal examination but even if your problem has nothing to do with that area he might carry out an acupuncture examination of the abdomen. This consists of very lightly feeling the surface of the tummy for changes in temperature which can give more information about the twelve internal organs. Areas of the abdomen 'reflect' different organs and this is illustrated in Table 11.

The practitioner will also carry out a normal physiological examination of the part of the body concerned. If you have a pain in the shoulder, for

TABLE 11

The front mu *or alarm points for each of the* zang fu. *These points are often spontaneously tender when there is an acute disorder of the related organ.*

ORGAN	ALARM POINT	APPROXIMATE LOCATION
Lungs	Zhongfu	Lower border of second rib on nipple line
Colon	Tianshu	Two thumbs' width each side of navel
Stomach	Zhongwang	Midway between navel and lower end of breast bone
Spleen	Zhangmen	Free end of eleventh rib
Heart	Jujue	On the midline eight fingers' width above the navel
Small intestines	Guanyuan	On the midline four fingers' width below the navel
Bladder	Zhongji	One thumb's width below guanyuan
Kidneys	Jingmen	Free end of twelfth rib
Three heater	Shimen	On midline two thumbs' width below the navel
Heart constrictor	Shanzhong	On the midline over the breast bone at the level of the nipples
Gall bladder	Riyue	Between 7th and 8th ribs on the nipple line
Liver	Qimen	Two intercostal spaces directly below the nipple.

example, he will test your shoulder by asking you to move your arm in different directions and then moving it for you to see if these 'passive' movements are easier for you. Finally, he will ask you to make the movements again but he will prevent you from actually carrying them out. This forces you to tighten your muscles without causing any movement and enables the doctor to find out if the problem is in the muscles or in the joint. He will also feel or palpate your shoulder to see if there is any swelling or inflammation.

Next, the acupuncturist might carry out some special tests using foot zone therapy or applied kinesiology (*see* chapter 10) or he might even make use of one of the currently available diagnostic instruments. However, no practitioner is likely to do all these things and he will have selected the methods which he can do best and which he feels are the most suitable. Do not, therefore, having read this book expect everything to be followed to the letter! More experienced acupuncturists are often able to make quite a rapid diagnosis with comparatively little testing. However, if your acupuncturist does not examine you at all you should certainly go elsewhere.

THE TREATMENT

The time will now have arrived for you to receive the first treatment. Your predominant question will probably be, 'Is it going to hurt?' The answer is that it should be hardly painful at all. Sometimes it is so painless that a patient will not realise that a needle has been inserted, but on other occasions there is a mild burning sensation rather like a slight bee sting. If strong stimulation is sought by the doctor, you will certainly feel something as the needle is manipulated, but this should be a sensation of numbness, heaviness or tingling rather than actual pain. As it is your first visit he will probably put no more than three or four needles in, but in subsequent visits this may be increased.

Although the acupuncturist will normally be only too pleased to talk about your problems and discuss the treatment with you he cannot concentrate on doing the acupuncture if he is being asked difficult questions at the same time — so try to keep these to a time before the treatment starts or after the needles have all been inserted. Anyway, by the time you have read this book you might be able to tell him what he is doing anyway!

The treatment can last from about five minutes up to half an hour and the average length of a session is about twenty minutes.

When the treatment is over, you will probably be wondering what it will do to you and how often you will have to have further treatments. To answer the first question, it will help to harmonise your body functions so that you will probably feel very relaxed and, possibly, light and springy when you walk out of the surgery. You might experience this feeling for just a few hours or maybe for the rest of the day. On the other hand you might feel very little or nothing at all. If it was a pain that took you along for the treatment it is very likely that it will already feel a little better. This lessening of the pain might last permanently or only for a short period of time. If it only lasts for a day or two or less, then you obviously require a few daily treatments or at least a few treatments on alternate days. As you get better, the treatments should be spaced out more. This has more or less answered the second question, but the total duration of the treatments or total number of treatments will depend upon the seriousness of your condition, the length of time you have had it and your own recuperative powers.

HERING'S LAW OF CURE

According to Constantine Hering, who was actually a homoeopath, a true cure takes place from the head downwards, from inside the body to the outside, from the more vital organs to the less vital and symptoms disappear in the reverse order to their appearance. The first part of Hering's Law implies that healing starts in the mind, but sometimes symptoms do in fact literally travel down the body on their way out. If a skin lesion occurs during treatment, this may very well be an indication that healing is taking place from inside out. The reappearance of long lost symptoms is a sure sign that healing is taking place. When symptoms change in reverse of Hering's Law we must ensure that they are not merely being suppressed and driven deeper into the body.

At this stage your acupuncturist might venture to give you some recommendations concerning your life style where a change would help you to be healthier. The ancient Chinese distinguished five levels of doctors. The lowest was the animal doctor who only treated animals. The next was the acupuncturist/herbalist who treated minor problems. The third level was the surgeon who treated more serious conditions. The fourth level was the nutritionist who taught people how to extend their lives and be healthier by eating correctly. The highest of all was the doctor who taught the 'laws of the universe' who could intuitively see how the patient was at variance with nature.

THE EIGHT PRINCIPLES

These are also known as the eight principal patterns of disharmony and form the basic diagnostic system of Traditional Chinese Medicine. The eight principles or categories are:

Yin	*Yang*
Cold	Hot
Internal	External
Deficiency	Excess

The categories of *yin* and *yang* have already been discussed in chapter 2, but Table 12 lists some common disorders in terms of their *yin/yang* predominance.

COLD AND HOT

A disease of cold is characterised by a dislike of cold, paleness, cold arms and legs or cold hands and feet, passing a lot of pale urine, thin white secretions, pain lessened by warmth, and having slow movements. The tongue is pale, swollen and with a white moss coating. There may be a desire to drink hot liquids and the patient may sleep curled up in bed.

A disease of heat is portrayed by quick, agitated movements, dislike of heat or hot weather, excessive thirst, desire for cold drinks, fever, constipation, small amounts of dark urine and a red tongue with a yellow moss. The pulse will be fast, whereas in the cold condition it is slow.

INTERNAL AND EXTERNAL

This is more or less self-explanatory. A skin problem, a common cold or a joint pain are external; whereas a generalised infection with high fever, inflammation of one of the organs or a growth or tumour inside the body are internal. Internal problems tend to be chronic and external ones acute.

DEFICIENCY AND EXCESS

These are generally coincident with *yin* and *yang*, though deficient *yang* and excess *yin* can also occur. Also, to complicate matters, it is possible to have two different types of condition co-existing. For example, an acute infection which is both hot and *yang* can be superimposed upon a chronic, cold, *yin* condition where there is frailty and general deficiency. (*See* Table 12.)

TABLE 12
Some common findings of ill-health classified in terms of yin *and* yang.

EXCESS YIN	EXCESS YANG
Self-conscious	Over-confident
Apathetic	Aggressive
Sad	Euphoric
Flabby muscles and tissue	Hard tissue/spastic muscles
Pale skin and complexion	Ruddy complexion
Slow metabolism	Fast metabolism
Weak pulse	Strong pulse
Slow speech/weak voice	Rapid speech/strong voice
Easily fatigued	Plenty of stamina
Low blood pressure	High blood pressure
Slow movements	Rapid movements

THE PULSE

The most important considerations regarding the pulse have already been mentioned, but as the pulse is such an important feature in the Chinese diagnostic system, a list of some of the pulse findings and their implications is given in Table 13.

TABLE 13
Some common pulse findings and their meanings.

PULSE	INTERPRETATION
Superficial pulse	Early stages of disease. Invasion of external pathogens
Deep pulse	Internal condition
Slow pulse	Cold syndrome
Rapid pulse	Hot syndrome
Weak pulse	Indicates deficiency
Strong pulse	Indicates excess
Intermittent pulse	Impairment of *qi* and blood
Wiry pulse	Insufficient liver *yin* and hyperactive liver *yang*
Knotted pulse	Cold phlegm and stagnant blood

SUMMARY

The causes of disease according to Chinese medicine are similar to those recognised by modern Western medicine but greater emphasis is placed upon the role of the spirit or mind which is thought to play a part in all diseases. The influence of adverse weather conditions is given greater recognition in the Chinese system. Diagnosis is made by taking a history, asking questions, observing the patient, examining relevant parts, looking at the complexion, ears, eyes, tongue and feeling the pulses. Testing for trigger points and alarm points and ascertaining any unusual odours are also important. The period of the day when the patient feels better or worse, unusual tastes in the mouth, food cravings, the nature of the voice, whether any type of weather or time of year influences the symptoms and the body type are all considered by the acupuncturist. It is also important that he is able to recognise the signs of good health because this helps in the identification of minor problems and imbalances.

6   *How the Treatment is Formulated*

So far, we have looked at the philosophy behind Chinese Medicine, how the Chinese described the formation of the body's energy and how it operates within the organism. We have noted how the energy may become disordered and how the acupuncturist can recognise this by his various diagnostic methods. Having made this diagnosis, how does the acupuncturist decide where, exactly, to put the needle?

LOCAL AND DISTAL POINTS

The acupuncturist's first consideration should be to give the patient relief from his symptoms, particularly if there is pain. For this he usually does local and distal points. This means that he treats points where the problem actually is or, in the case of referred pain, where the problem originates. Usually, one meridian is involved and the points will be selected from that meridian. In cases of shoulder pain, where five or six meridians pass close to one another, points may be selected from more than one meridian. Next, the acupuncturist will treat spontaneously sensitive points, which the Chinese call *ah shi* points, from the expression commonly used when these points are pressed. Many English students have held a quite erroneous belief about the origin of these words! The distal points are given in Table 14, but these are only the commonest ones. If possible, a distal point on the meridian being treated should be selected. The point *hegu* on the hand is often chosen in painful conditions since it is also a special point for pain. Thus, for facial pain it would serve the dual purpose of distal point and special point. The next most useful point for pain lies on the stomach meridian, on the foot between the second and third toes. This is also a distal point and is used particularly for pain in the lower half of the body. Sometimes, the end point, which might be the first or last point on the meridian, is used as a distal point. This is why, in acupuncture, we often treat a patient at the opposite end of the body. A patient, surprised that he had been given needles in his foot for pain in his head asked the nurse why this was. The nurse thought for a moment and said, 'It's like inflation, it starts low down but gradually works upwards!'

TABLE 14

The principal distal points and the areas which they cover.

DISTAL POINT	LOCATION	AREA AFFECTED
Hegu	Hand	Face, special sense organs, front of head and neck
Lieque	Wrist	Back of head, neck, back of chest and lungs
Neiguan	Arm	Front of chest, upper abdomen, internal organs of chest and upper abdomen, diaphragm
Zusanli	Leg	Internal organs of abdomen, especially intestines
Weizhong	Back of knee	Low back. Genito-urinary problems
Sanyinjiao	Leg	Crutch, pelvic organs and external sex organs

An example of the many cases where this approach is appropriate and successful was that of Mrs S.C. who first attended for acupuncture at the age of 47 with arthritis of the right hip of several years' duration. This lady had been advised to have a hip replacement and wanted to try acupuncture to see if she could obtain relief from her pain whilst she was waiting for surgery. She realised, of course, that acupuncture could not cure her and in her case the relief of symptoms was not only paramount but the only thing that could sensibly be done. A needle was inserted at the point near the hip which is known to be effective for hip pain and sciatica. A distal point influential for muscle and tendon was also used. Moxibustion, using the osteoarthritis technique of burning a small piece of moxa on the handle of the needle, was given to the first point and the patient reported complete relief from her symptoms after the third treatment. By a process of trial and error she discovered that the effect of the treatment lasted for about three months and at regular quarterly intervals returned for a 'top up'. This continued with amazing regularity for some five years until she moved to a distant part of the country and was given a new practitioner. During these years Mrs C. had not only been pain free but had been able to postpone her hip replacement which is very helpful in a fairly young person. It should also be recorded that this lady, apart from her arthritic hip, which was brought on by an accident, was very fit and had no apparent signs of any other problems.

The use of local and distal points incorporates two fundamentals of acupuncture: that all acupuncture points treat diseases of the local and surrounding areas, and that all acupuncture points treat diseases occurring along the meridian as well as those of the pertaining organ, related tissue and connected organ of special sense (*see* Table 15). In this particular case we were able to use the gall bladder meridian which passed over the area of

TABLE 15
The influential points.

INFLUENTIAL POINT	TISSUE
Shanzong	Respiratory system
Dashu	Bone and cartilage
Geshu	Blood
Zhongwan	*Fu* (The hollow, '*yang*' organs)
Zhangmen	*Zang* (The solid, '*yin*' organs)
Taiyuan	Vascular system
Yanglingquan	Muscle and tendons
Xuanzhong	Bone marrow

trouble and has as its related tissue the muscles and ligaments. Local, distal and *ah shi* points combine three different methods of employing acupuncture points and these are frequently used together.

POINTS WITH SPECIAL EFFECTS

a) *Analgesia* Acupuncture is a powerful analgesic and the most effective analgesic points have already been mentioned.

b) *Sedation* There are a number of points which have a specifically sedative effect; particularly *baihui* on the head, *shenmen* on the wrist, *hegu* on the hand, *fenglong* on the leg, *yanglingquan* on the leg and *taichong* on the foot. One or more of these points or pairs of points are usually combined with other points, though sometimes where the condition being treated is nervousness or anxiety they may be used alone.

c) *Homoeostasis* This means the tendency to maintain balance within the body. Some points have a particularly homeostatic effect and help to regulate temperature, respiration, heart rate, sleep, appetite, muscle tone, acid-alkali balance, endocrine secretions, regularity of movement and secretions of the digestive tract, etc. The best points for this are *quchi* at the elbow, *zusanli* on the leg and *sanyinjiao* on the inside of the leg.

d) *Immune Enhancing Points* Acupuncture has been used for thousands of years by the Chinese in the treatment of infection and it has been shown that certain points have a considerable effect in raising the body's defence mechanisms. The most effective of these are *dazhui* on the neck, *quchi*, *zusanli* and *sanyinjiao*.

e) *Motor Effects*   These are points which are situated over the main motor-points of the body which are associated with the gross motor muscles. These points are used in cases of paralysis or muscular weakness. Treatment using these points has been successfully employed in cases of poliomyelitis particularly in India.

THE INFLUENTIAL POINTS

There are eight influential points which have a special action on the specific tissues to which they are related. These are listed in Table 15.

THE *Xi*-CLEFT POINTS

There is one *xi*-cleft point on each of the main meridians and these points are particularly effective in the treatment of acute conditions which are either associated with the meridian or its pertaining organ. An acute cough, for example, was treated by using the *xi*-cleft point on the lung meridian. *Xi*-cleft points can be remarkably effective when correctly chosen.

THE *MU* (ALARM) AND *SHU* (ORGAN ASSOCIATED) POINTS

The front *mu* points have already been described in chapter 5 and are listed in Table 11. When used in treatment they are quite often combined with the back *shu* points: though either may be used independently. The back *shu* points are points on the bladder meridian which are situated each side of the vertebrae from the third thoracic down to the sacrum. They relate to the outflow of the sympathetic ganglia which contribute nerves from each spinal segment to the various internal organs. These points are undoubtedly influenced by deep massage and vertebral manipulation which is carried out by osteopaths. This is another way of explaining some of the effects of osteopathy. In acupuncture the points are treated in the usual way with needles. Moxibustion may also be applied with or without needles. Generally, acupuncturists use a toning or stimulating technique on these points as they are in direct contact with the organs. However, 'perverse' energy, which we have avoided discussing up until now, may be drawn off at these points. Perverse energy can be considered as one or other of the external disease factors which gain access to the body when the defensive energy is weak and upset the normal vibratory frequencies. It is only when this disorder reaches one of the organs that its related *shu* points would be used to calm or remove it. The *shu* points lie about one and a half thumbs' width either side of the vertebral column. The same distance away laterally is another series of points which correspond to the same organs on a spiritual or emotional level and would be used for shock, excessive grief or any disease which had its origin in such emotional trauma.

A young girl of 14 who was suffering from anorexia nervosa, which dated from the death of her pet rabbit, responded very well to acupuncture in which these points were used.

THE FIVE ELEMENTS

Points may be selected on the basis of imbalances found in the five elements, sometimes called transformations or phases. Using the Mother-Son Law, a deficiency would be treated by enhancing the transfer of energy from the 'mother' organ on the *sheng* cycle. For example, a deficiency found in the kidney could be treated by drawing energy from the lungs (*see* Figure 4). Because the lungs are related to the element 'metal' the metal point on the kidney meridian would be used for treatment. The yang *(fu)* organs can be dealt with in the same way. Sometimes the influence of the *ko* cycle can be made use of and in the case of kidney deficiency this may be because too great an inhibitory influence is being exerted by the spleen (earth). In addition, there may be overactivity of the heart which is not being controlled by water. The precise treatment would depend upon the exact findings but it is possible that the 'earth' point of the kidneys might be used.

A good example of the use of the five elements was that of Miss N.T. who was suffering from chronic constipation and sinusitis. The colon was found to be deficient and the simple expedient of treating the earth point *quchi* at the elbow was remarkably effective. Additional relief for the head problems was obtained by deep pressure massage on the points *fengchi* on the gall bladder meridian at the back of the skull. These points are known to be effective in the treatment of many kinds of headache and 'fuzziness' in the head.

In cases of migraine, an imbalance of energy is often found between the liver and gall bladder and there is often an overactive state of these organs. Although one has to be very careful when treating the heart meridian, good results are sometimes achieved by merely treating the point *shaochong* at the tip of the little finger, for this is the wood point of the heart meridian and encourages the transfer of energy from liver to heart. Professor Jayasuriya was one of the first to do this particular treatment as previously most practitioners had used points on the liver or gall bladder or heart constrictor meridians.

Horary points may be used in conformity with the Chinese clock and this has already been described in chapter 3.

THE EIGHT EXTRA MERIDIANS

These meridians are used for treatment, mostly by using what are known as the 'key' or 'confluent' points. These are pairs of points, each pair being used to bring into play one of the meridians. Two pairs of key points are normally used together, so that two of the extra meridians are employed. The normal coupling of the points, the meridians which they control and the indications for use are given in Table 16.

THE EIGHT DIAGNOSTIC PRINCIPLES

As a result of a diagnosis utilising the eight diagnostic principles, points may be used for their known energic influences. In Table 17, some patterns of

TABLE 16
The extra meridians, key points and areas and symptoms which they cover.

KEY POINT	EXTRA MERIDIAN	AREA OF BODY AND INDICATIONS
Neiguan	Yin Wei Mo (Yin Energy Conserver)	Heart, chest and stomach. Nervousness, varicose veins, pain in chest, timidity, indigestion, abdominal pain, amnesia,
Gongsun	Chong Mo (Vital Energy Regulator)	hyperacidity, heart disease, palpitations, gastric ulcers.
Houxi	Du mo (Governor)	Neck, shoulder, back and inner corner of eyes.
Shenmai	Yang Chiao Mo (Yang Energy Accelerator)	Epilepsy, febrile disease, articulatory and locomotor problems, insomnia, paranoia, obsessional neurosis, manic-depressive state, hormonal imbalance.
Waiguan	Yang Wei Mo (Yang Energy Conserver)	Area behind ears, outer corner of eyes and cheeks. Coldness, arthritis of toes, acne, boils, earache, chills, fever, tinnitus, toothache,
Foot Linqi	Dai Mo (Belt Channel)	abdominal distension, weakness and motor impairment in the lumbar region.
Lieque	Ren Mo (Conception Vessel)	Throat, chest & lungs. Asthma, bronchitis, epilepsy, eczema, headache, hay fever,
Zhaohai	Yin Chiao Mo (Yin Energy Accelerator)	laryngitis, sore throat, urino-genital disorders, sexual weakness, difficult birth, cystitis, sleepiness, toxaemia of pregnancy, post partum pains and bleeding, bladder weakness.

disharmony are listed, together with the related signs and symptoms, and the Western medical equivalents. As there are a large number of such patterns which are not listed, it is not felt appropriate to indicate the actual points which might be used and in any case these would vary in individual cases.

JUNCTION POINTS

These are the junction points between the meridians of coupled organs which are heart and small intestines, spleen and stomach, lung and colon, kidney and bladder, liver and gall bladder and heart constrictor and three heater. These points are used particularly when there is an imbalance between any two organ pairs as they activate the joining vessels. These points are normally used in conjunction with the source or *yuan* points. The use of junction points could be considered to be a subcategory of the use of the five phases.

MODERN MEDICINE

Although not a desirable method in the author's opinion, acupuncture points may be selected merely in terms of the doctor's understanding of the patient's problem in terms of Western medicine. This is a 'hit and miss' affair because Western medicine takes little or no cognisance of the individuality of the patient and focuses its attention almost exclusively on the disease *per se*. For example, there are at least four different patterns of disharmony associated with bronchial asthma, two of which are illustrated in Table 17; yet Western medicine would regard them all as the same disease. Moreover, the acupuncturist will recognise nuances of energy disturbance even within those four major patterns and his treatment will be exactly tailored to the patient at every stage of his progress back to health. The Western medical approach could be even more misleading in this instance because of its preoccupation with the site of manifestation of the disease which is the lungs, rather than the *origin* of the disease which may be in the digestive system. This is a fact that has always been insisted upon by naturopaths and is in conformity with the five elements where earth (digestion) is the 'mother' or nourisher of the metal (respiration).

AURICULAR ACUPUNCTURE

This is a specialised form of acupuncture where the treatment is carried out on points on the external ear. This part of the ear is endowed with points which reflexly affect every part of the body (*see* Figure 9) and these points

TABLE 17

A few examples of patterns of disharmony in terms of Chinese medicine, the signs and symptoms and equivalent designation in Western medicine.

PATTERNS IN CHINESE MEDICINE	OBSERVATIONS AND SYMPTOMS	WESTERN EQUIVALENT
Hyperactive liver *yang*. Retention of damp phlegm	Vertigo, tinnitus, nausea, red tongue and wiry, rapid pulse. Fullness and suffocating sensation of chest, nausea and vomiting, white sticky moss on tongue. Slippery pulse.	Hypertension
Deficient *qi* and blood	Lassitude, palpitation, insomnia, weak pulse.	
Wind-cold of lung	Cough with thin sputum, shortness of breath, white moss on tongue, superficial pulse.	Bronchial asthma
Phlegm-heat of lungs	Rapid and coarse breathing. Thick purulent sputum, thick, yellow moss on tongue and rapid pulse.	
Insufficient kidney *yang*	Pallor, dizziness, blurred vision, listlessness, lumbar soreness, frequency of urination, thready pulse.	Impotence
Wind obstructing meridians	Sore, painful joints. Pain moves around. White moss on tongue.	Arthritis
Cold obstructing meridians	Painful joints, worse with movement. Pain does not move. Worse in cold.	
Damp heat obstructing meridians	Swollen and painful joints. Fever and thirst. Tongue reddish with greasy, yellow moss. Rapid pulse.	Rheumatoid arthritis

may be needled in conformity with the accepted rules of acupuncture. For example, a person suffering from an eye disorder might have needles placed in the 'eye' points of the ear, together with liver and gall bladder points, which are couple organs of the related element (*see* Table 5). The point of the bladder might be included on account of the close proximity of the bladder meridian to the eye.

A good illustration of the powerful effect of auricular acupuncture is illustrated by the case of Mr P.K. who was a young man of twenty-five suffering from severe pain in the penis whenever having an erection. He had received a variety of treatments including acupuncture, and was in a state of despair. His acupuncturist advised him to have auricular acupuncture but, not doing it himself, left the lad to find another practitioner. He ended up in

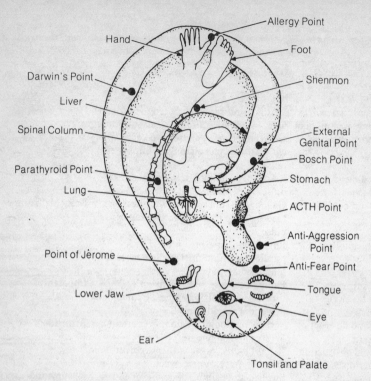

Figure 9 Some of the more commonly used acupuncture points found on the ear. Darwin's point is used for treating sleep disturbances; the Bosch point is used for psychosexual disorders; the allergy point is used for allergic conditions; and shenmen is used for emotional or nervous problems. The point of Jerome is also used for relaxation purposes, and to treat sleep problems.

my surgery and the situation more or less obliged me to treat him with auriculotherapy, even though my experience of it at that time was very little. He was treated principally with the external genital point and a press needle (*see* next chapter) was placed on this point and retained by the patient who was instructed to press on it every day and at any time he experienced the pain. Ten days later he reported a considerable improvement and about a week after his second treatment telephoned my office to say that he was 'completely cured' and would like to cancel his next appointment as it entailed a long and difficult journey. It seemed almost too good to be true because this boy had been suffering for seven years, but quite by coincidence the author met him two years later at an exhibition and he reported two years of complete freedom from his problem. It scarcely seems necessary to relate how grateful he was!

Auriculotherapy is an ancient form of treatment and was doubtless effective because the ear is richly endowed with nerves which have connections all over the body. This form of treatment has received a great deal of attention in modern times and Dr Nogier from France is mentioned in the Appendix. In Germany the Munich Auriculotherapy Association has more than 3,000 members which is an indication of the popularity and widespread use of this form of acupuncture.

Each cell in the body carries within its chromosomes a computer-like representation of all the features of the entire body and this is probably the theoretical basis for these various reflex areas. Moreover, the entire body can be superimposed on the ear (*see* Figure 9) and it is found that different parts of the ear are embryologically connected with the corresponding areas of the body superimposed upon them. Since 1966 auriculotherapy has been widely used all over China for both treatment and anaesthesia. It has been found most useful for disorders of the internal organs and may be combined with body acupuncture or other forms of acupuncture.

SCALP, NOSE, HAND, FOOT, WRIST AND ANKLE ACUPUNCTURE

Apart from the regular points which occur on the head, hands and feet, these areas, as well as the nose, serve as reflex areas to the entire body in a similar way to the ears.

SCALP

Scalp or head acupuncture is based upon areas of the scalp which are related to the motor areas of the cortex of the brain. These areas were mapped out by Jiao Shen-fa, a neurologist in the Ji Shan People's Hospital in the Shanshi Province of the People's Republic of China, during the time of the Cultural Revolution (1966-69). Shen-fa, who also had a good knowledge of acupuncture, took to heart the exhortation of Chairman Mao for physicians of both traditional and modern disciplines to put aside their political differences and work together for the benefit of the people, and he started work on a case of hemiplegia (one sided paralysis) by stimulating with a needle the area on the scalp which corresponded to the motor area of the cortex. The results were astonishing: the patient experienced a sensation in the paralysed limbs during the treatment and afterwards had a greater degree of movement in them. After Shen-fa had reported his findings, other workers established many other areas on the scalp relating to different cortical functions. Usually, the scalp area is situated fairly close to the corresponding part of the cerebral cortex, but the connection is an electro-physiological one rather than being strictly topographical. Since the measurement of electrical activity in the brain is regularly made on the scalp in Western medical practice when an electro-encephalogram is recorded, this phenomena should be readily understood by Western trained scientists. Conditions most frequently treated by scalp acupuncture are paralysis, mental disorders, speech disorders, cardiovascular problems and genito-urinary disorders.

NOSE
Nose or 'Face-Nose' acupuncture is similar to ear acupuncture in that there are points on the nose which relate to different areas of the body. As in ear acupuncture, the needle should only be inserted superficially and always on the outside or external part.

FOOT AND HAND
In the case of the foot and hand, points may be treated with a needle or massaged. The author is opposed to placing needles on the under-surface of the foot and feels that this is an area which should be given massage only. The reflex areas on the foot are shown in Figure 10. The reflexes on the hand or foot should be treated with a deep compression massage.

WRIST-ANKLE
Wrist-ankle acupuncture is a comparatively new technique which started after a paper was published by the Department of Neurology of the First Teaching Hospital of the Second Army Medical College in Shanghai, People's Republic of China, in 1976. This new form of acupuncture was developed because the wrist and ankle are less sensitive areas than the hand or foot. The method is easy to learn and simple to use and is economical in terms of needles which is a consideration always relevant in the Third World. Moreover, the therapeutic results are very good. There are twelve points, six at the wrist and six at the ankle, and the needle is inserted just under the skin in a horizontal fashion. The needle is not manipulated and is retained in the position for about 20-30 minutes. The method has proved to be very effective in acute disorders such as sore throat, headaches, toothache,

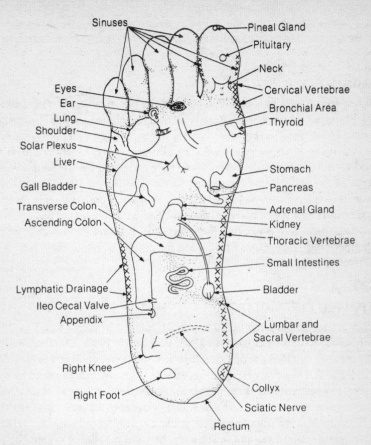

Figure 10 The right foot showing the acupuncture micro-system which is commonly termed foot reflexology. These reflexes may become simultaneously sensitive with a disorder in the part of the body to which they are related. Treatment to the reflex is usually done with a deep, compression type of massage and is often known as foot zone therapy.

low back pain, neuralgia, menstrual pain and pain in the limbs. If the pain is in the hand or foot, the needle is directed towards the site of pain: in all other cases it is directed towards the elbow or knee according to whether it has been inserted at the wrist or ankle. Very good results have also been obtained with this technique in cases of nasal discharge, bronchial asthma, allergic inflammation of the gut, incontinence of urine, and leucorrhoea (vaginal discharge); whilst fairly good results have been noted in stroke cases, insomnia, disturbances of sensation, hypertension, and mental disorders.

IRIDOLOGY

Reflex areas have also been found in the iris, a phenomenon first noticed by Dr Philippus Meyens in 1670. It was later developed by the Hungarian doctor Ignatz von Peczely who, as a boy of ten, noticed the appearance of a dark stripe in the iris of an owl that had broken its leg. Later, as a medical student and as a doctor he began to correlate regions in the iris with specific areas of the body and first published his findings in 1866. Since then numerous physicians have elaborated the theme and iridology or iris diagnosis is now a well accepted diagnostic science. We do not use the eyes for treatment purposes, but the diagnostic information which can be obtained from the eyes may be used to formulate the treatment which will ultimately be given.

APPLIED KINESIOLOGY

This is another system which has been developed in recent times and the only one to have originated in the USA. In the early 1960s, Dr Goodheart, a chiropractor, noticed a connection between muscle function and organs. He was led to this discovery because, in defiance of mainstream thought, he was trying to find methods of strengthening weak muscles instead of endlessly ironing out spastic ones which would inevitably tighten up after the treatment. Having discovered that muscles could be affected by related acupuncture meridians and, ultimately, by their pertaining organs, he set about finding ways to strengthen weak muscles and in doing so borrowed the acupuncture points known as Chapman's reflexes and one or two other useful methods of treatment. The reflex points used were renamed 'neurovascular' and 'neurolymphatic' points in conformity with their activity which was to enhance the blood supply or lymphatic drainage respectively. All these points are extremely well illustrated in *Touch for Health* by Dr John Tie and Mary Marks. Since Goodheart's discovery the principle has been extensively researched and an entire diagnostic system formulated in which subtle changes in muscle function can be used to diagnose functional disorders and energy imbalances. The method can be used for testing the presence of allergens, undesirable foods, poisons, medication, vitamins and food supplements and it is even possible to use it to test the suitability of a proposed treatment. Some problems, such as ionisation disorders, can scarcely be found by any other method.

THROUGH AND THROUGH ACUPUNCTURE

In this method, two or more points are joined up by the insertion of the needle. The selection of points is made on the basis of the special therapeutic property of the combined points.

7 *The Needles*

In the early days of acupuncture needles were made from pieces of stone or flint and in 1926 several quartz needles were excavated at Chou Kou Tien near Peking. Bamboo needles were also certainly used as the ancient Chinese ideograph for 'needle' incorporated the idea of bamboo and only in later years did this become altered to imply metal. Bronze, stone and bone needles were all unearthed in 1899 at Hsiao, Tun Yuan Shui, An Yang County, Honan Province. According to Chuang Yu-Min, carapace needles usually made from turtle shells were used in acupuncture treatment as early as three thousand years ago, and the stone needles from An Yang were dated from about 1700 BC.

These early stone needles were called *bian* which actually means using stone to treat disease. In the late Neolithic period around 2000 BC, ceramic needles were introduced and by about 1600 BC in the Bronze Age metal needles were first manufactured. It was not until the Warring States period (403-221 BC) that advances in metallurgy made it possible to manufacture fine, steel needles which were ideally suited to the practice of acupuncture. Although gold and silver needles were thought to be superior – and still are by the French – the consensus of opinion is that the modern, stainless steel acupuncture needle is second to none.

Traditionally, nine varieties of needle were used and these may be summarised as:

1 The *arrowhead needle* used for drawing blood and treating hot conditions.
2 The *round needle* used for rubbing against the skin and treating stagnant *qi*.
3 The *pressure needle* which had a tip shaped like a grain of millet and was used for shallow treatment of meridians.
4 The *sharp needle* which was round with a sharp tip and used to drain abscesses.
5 The *sword needle* which was similar to the sharp needle but larger and used for draining superficial abscesses.

6   The *round-sharp* needle which had a thin, round body and slightly expanded head and was used for elimination of obstruction.

7   The *fine, filiform needle* which had a thin shaft and was used for the elimination of cold, heat, pain and obstruction.

8   The *long needle*, similar to the previous type but longer and used for deep insertion.

9   The *large needle* which had a thick body and was used for the treatment of arthritis and draining fluids.

Needles in present day use are a little different to the ancient needles and are as follows:

1   *The filiform needle.* This is the commonest type of needle used in acupuncture and the only type used by some practitioners. The shaft is made of stainless steel and the handle has a superimposition of copper, bronze, silver or stainless steel. By having a different metal on the handle there will be differential heating when moxa is applied to the needle and this results in a tiny electrical discharge which runs down the needle. Whether or not this influences treatment is still open to argument. The length of the needles varies from 12.7mm to 203.2mm. Occasionally, even longer needles are used and these may be threaded down the back to join up a whole series of points. The diameter of the needles varies from 0.46mm to as little as 0.19mm and the following table shows different gauges in general use.

Gauge	26	28	30	32	34
Diameter (mm)	0.46	0.38	0.32	0.26	0.23

Gauge and corresponding diameter in mm of the commonly used acupuncture needles.

Thirty or thirty-two gauge needles are usually selected for acupuncture on the face and around the eyes, for children or cases where very little stimulation is required. If longer needles are used a wider gauge is usually chosen and wider gauge needles are needed for a treatment requiring strong stimulation. The most popular needle is the 38.1mm 28 gauge which might be considered an 'all purpose' needle.

2   *The embedding needle.* This is also called the press needle, intradermal

71

needle or implanted needle. Its purpose is to be inserted and left *in situ*. The commonest design is the thumbtack type which is 2-3mm long and has a small circular head at right angles to the shaft. The head prevents entry of the entire needle. It is most frequently used for ear acupuncture and may be pressed from time to time when in position – hence the name 'press' needle. Another variety is a tiny stainless steel ball which is applied to the acupuncture point with adhesive. This is not strictly a needle and cannot be inserted through the skin. It is safer than the needle and is more pleasant for the patient. The most recent innovation is a squarer design of the ball-bearing type which is magnetised. These are now under research and it is too early to say if they are superior to non-magnetised needles.

There are other designs of embedding needles, most of which are longer than the thumbtack type and these are used for embedding in acupuncture points on the body.

3 *The plum blossom needle.* This is also known as the 'five star' or 'seven star' needle. It consists of five or seven short needles protruding from a holder which is attached to a long handle. This instrument is used to tap along the meridians or on specific areas of skin and is used on children, weak or elderly patients, for skin conditions and for those patients who dislike puncturing or who are allergic to needles.

4 *The hot needle.* This needle is fairly thick in gauge and is made from a special alloy of silver. It is brought to red heat and plunged into certain types of superficial swellings or ganglions. The needle is immediately withdrawn so that it only remains in contact with the flesh for a fraction of a second.

5 *The prismatic needle.* This is a needle with a triangular point and is used to induce bleeding at certain points. This treatment is mostly used for certain types of inflammatory conditions, acute disturbances and allergic skin conditions.

6 *Rolling drum.* This is really a variation of the plum blossom needle. It consists of a revolving drum with rows of protruding needles which can be 'run' up and down the skin over a meridian.

STERILIZATION OF NEEDLES

Needles have to be sterilized, particularly after being used. Some needles are

72

pre-sterilized and disposable but are mostly not very suitable for acupuncture as the practitioner cannot get the full feed-back through the handle; nor can he manipulate them easily. A standard type of pre-sterilized needle has now been produced by Acumedic in the UK and these are quite satisfactory for acupuncture use. Moreover, if desired, they can be sterilized after treatment and re-used. Other needles should be fully sterilized before being used, though cleansing with surgical spirit is probably quite satisfactory.

Once a needle has been used for a treatment it must be discarded or sterilized by autoclaving or an equivalent process. After removal, the needle should be cleansed by wiping with surgical spirit or a dilute antiseptic. It should then be autoclaved and subsequently retained in a closed container until required again. The skin is usually swabbed with alcohol before needle insertion, but this does not seem to be necessary. It is important that the doctor's fingers are scrupulously clean when carrying out acupuncture. Infections being transmitted by acupuncture treatment are almost unheard of but there was a single case of an unqualified practitioner in England who managed to spread serum hepatitis because of his lack of training and ignorance of correct sterilization. Since then, local authorities in Britain have attempted to control the practice of acupuncture to minimise the possibility of any repetition of such an event, but no member of the public need have any qualms about this aspect of acupuncture if the practitioner is a properly qualified and registered acupuncturist.

Needles should not be repeatedly re-used as they tend to become pitted and blunted and the metal tends to get fatigued with repeated sterilizing. This means that the treatment is likely to be more painful than it should and there is a risk of the needle breaking after being inserted. After ten years of practice and thousands of acupuncture treatments the author has yet to see this happen; so one can rest assured that it is a rare occurrence. Usually it can easily be dealt with by a qualified practitioner.

METHODS OF INSERTION

Acupuncturists do not just push needles into bodies in the way that doctors and nurses give hypodermic injections. Apart from the fact that the point, which is less than a millimetre in diameter, has to be carefully located, the angle and depth of insertion vary at each point and have to be correctly observed. Some points are needled perpendicularly to the skin surface; many are needled at an angle of about 45 degrees and some are needled almost

73

horizontally with the needle making an angle of 15 to 25 degrees with the skin.

Needles should be inserted rapidly through the outer layers of tissue in order to make the operation as painless as possible. From then onwards, the way in which the needle is introduced depends upon the type of treatment desired. In any event the acupuncturist aims to obtain a sensation (felt by the patient!) which is termed *deqi*. This is a sensation of either numbness, tingling, heaviness, soreness, distension or a feeling of slight pain at a distance from the site of puncture. Frequently, *deqi* is felt as a radiating sensation and experienced along the acupuncture meridian. Considerable research on this sensation has been carried out in recent years in the People's Republic of China and a paper was read at a World Congress on Acupuncture by Professor Zhu Zong Xiang of the Institute of Biophysics of the Chinese Academy of Sciences, Beijing (Peking) in which he described how he had traced out a sensitive line on the body by combining electrical and mechanical stimuli. 'This line', he said, 'was coincident with the classical channel course known by all acupuncturists.' He called this the 'latent propagating sensation along channel' (LPSC). 'LPSC', he stated, 'may be induced almost on everybody at any of the twelve main channels.' On the other hand, the propagating sensation along channel (PSC) is not frequently met in acupuncture clinics but is a more prominent sensation. Professor Zong Xiang concluded that 'LPSC which coincides with the classical channel is a general, physiological meridian phenomenon' and that the 'meridian system is realistically existent'.

Deqi may also be picked up by the acupuncturist and is recognisable as a sense of tightening felt through the needle handle which results from local muscle spasm in the patient. Some acupuncturists claim to be able to feel a subtle sensation on the hand when it is held at a distance from the needle, but this cannot yet be agreed as an objective, reproduceable phenomenon. Research in China has shown that acupuncturist's *deqi* is not felt if a muscle has lost its nerve supply.

Different qualities of *deqi* are usually obtained in different areas. Where the muscle mass is thin the feeling is usually that of local distension, whereas if the muscle is thick it is usually one of numbness or soreness. If the acupuncture point is close to a nerve trunk, the sensation is likely to be that of tingling or 'electric shock'. In some instances *deqi* cannot be obtained and this does not mean that the treatment is not working. It must be stressed that *deqi* although not pleasant is quite distinct from the sensation of pain.

The following techniques are some of those which may be used by acupuncturists to 'manipulate' the needle immediately after insertion:

1   *Raising and thrusting.* In this technique the needle is thrust up and down by a push-pull force exerted on the handle. The correct depth should first be obtained by prescience or *deqi* (or both!) and the needle then lifted just a few millimetres and immediately returned to the original depth. The amplitude of the movement may be increased for very strong stimulation, but the needle should on no account be completely withdrawn. If *deqi* is not obtained the angle of the return thrust may be very slightly varied with a view to seeking an elusive point.

2   *Twirling or rotating.* In this case the needle is introduced to the correct depth as before but is then rotated by approximately 180 degrees. This is usually repeated for about half a minute, allowing the needle to return to neutral more or less by itself. According to tradition, if the needle is rotated clockwise it invokes a stimulating process and if anti-clockwise it causes sedation.

3   *Combination of raising and thrusting with rotation.* This is a more difficult manoeuvre to perform but generally gives better results. It is also thought

TABLE 18
The classical procedures of bu *(stimulation) used mainly for* yin *disorders, and* xie *(calming) used chiefly for* yang *disorders.*

BU (Stimulation)	XIE (Calming)
Massage point before and after needling	Do not massage
Use gold needle	Use silver needle
Insert at end of expiration	Insert during inhalation
Insert obliquely in direction of energy flow	Insert obliquely against direction of energy flow
Insert rapidly	Insert slowly
Rotate clockwise	Rotate anticlockwise
Manipulate for a few seconds	Do not manipulate or manipulate for several minutes
Withdraw immediately	Retain for 10-12 minutes
Withdraw slowly during inhalation	Withdraw rapidly during exhalation
Close exit (by finger pressure)	Leave exit open

that by thrusting the needle during the patient's out-breath and raising or lifting during an inspiration a greater degree of stimulation is obtained and, conversely, by introducing the needle during the inspiratory phase and withdrawing it during expiration a greater degree of sedation is brought about. Manual manipulation to induce analgesia has to be done fairly rapidly and has to be sustained for the duration of surgery. Except for dental extraction which is almost instantaneous, electrical stimulation is used during surgery as it is more reliable, less tiring and more acceptable to the patient. The classical procedures are summarised in Table 18, but are not frequently used by modern acupuncturists. It can be seen from this table that the length of needle retention is also thought to influence the degree of stimulation or sedation, but this becomes very confusing since over-stimulation results in sedation and the cycle of stimulation-sedation-stimulation is repetitive.

4   *Other techniques.* These include:

a)   Plucking. In this case the needle head is 'flicked' by the operator's index finger.

b)   Scraping. The needle is held firmly with one hand whilst the fingernail of the index finger of the other hand is rubbed up and down the handle, sending a vibration down the entire needle.

c)   Trembling. This is a similar technique to that of raising and thrusting but the amplitude is so small that the effect is a vibration or trembling of the needle.

Before puncturing, it is important for the physician to select the correct needles and these should be approximately twice the length of the depth of insertion. This permits good manipulation of the needle and avoids the risk of placing the needle to its full depth, which should *never* happen under any circumstances. The needle may also be influenced with electricity or heat and these techniques will be explained in the following two chapters.

GENERAL TECHNIQUES OF NEEDLING
The specific techniques of needling will not be dealt with in this book since they are more of interest to the practitioner than the general reader. This also

refs to the positioning of the patient which must be both comfortable and appropriate for the particular treatment which is to take place.

The order of inserting and removing needles is important since it reflects the general rule that one should be orderly in one's activities. The general rule is to treat from above downwards but it is also in order to treat painful areas or lesions before other points.

Some acupuncturists have taken the question of sterility to ridiculous extremes by using the so-called 'no touch' method of needle insertion. To do this the needle is handled only with sterilised forceps and is never touched by the fingers until it has been fully inserted. This technique is valuable where very deep penetration is desired, but would seem to be quite unnecessary and even counter-productive in other cases since it renders the appreciation of feedback from the needle impossible and negates the basic principle of acupuncture.

The final word on needling should rest with Professor Jayasuriya who writes in his *Text Book of Acupuncture Science*, 'When the acupuncturist has learnt to needle little children satisfactorily he can indeed claim to have reached proficiency in the art of needling'.

TABLE 19
Methods of needle stimulation most often in use today

TYPE OF STIMULUS	METHOD	EFFECT	INDICATION
Strong	Needle is rotated, raised and thrust rapidly with a good amplitude	Sensation is strong with wide propagation along meridian	Patients with strong constitutions. For acute pain, cramps and Excess conditions
Mild	Needle is rotated, raised and thrust slowly with small amplitude	Slight sensation not usually propagated	Weak or nervous patients, those with history of fainting. For Deficient conditions
Moderate	Between strong and mild methods	Moderate sensation which may extend along meridian	Used in most cases

77

8 *The Scientific Explanation for Acupuncture*

When acupuncture was introduced to the West, those who had been brought up in the Western medical tradition naturally wanted to be able to explain it in terms with which they were already familiar. Moreover, scientific medicine looked askance at a method of treatment which it was unable to understand or explain. Consequently, many theories and some facts were established and these will be summarised in this chapter. Most of the following theories have a good deal of truth in them and each has a contribution to make towards the full understanding of the subject. However, it has to be reiterated that we are dealing with the very basic stuff of life and this has always proved elusive to the penetration of the scientific approach. In the end, it may have to be confessed that we cannot entirely place acupuncture within the framework of scientific medicine, not because it is unscientific but because it contains principles and truths which the human mind itself has difficulty grappling with. Neither the concept of God nor the *Tao* can be encompassed within the scientific models and acupuncture may be partly in the same category. Meanwhile, some answers have been provided and these may help our understanding of acupuncture: equally, by obscuring traditional thought it might lead us into further misunderstanding and this depends on the attitude of mind of the enquirer.

THE NEURAL THEORY

Put in the simplest form possible this theory maintains that pressure or irritation on the acupuncture point transmits 'repair' messages to the brain which are relayed to the centre which monitors body repair and mobilises the appropriate mechanisms.

This process involves what is known as the cutaneo-visceral reflex. The phenomenon was first noted in the West by the British neurologist Henry Head, and subsequently formulated in Head's Law which states that, 'When a painful stimulus is applied to a part of low sensibility in close central connection with a part of much greater sensibility, the pain produced is felt in the part of higher sensibility rather than in the part of lower sensibility to which the stimulus was actually applied'. This is a rather long-winded way of saying that a dysfunction in an organ of the body can be manifested on an area of skin which is either painful or unduly sensitive. Every organ has a related area of skin which lies adjacent or fairly near to it. Inflammation of the stomach is reflected in the adbominal area above the navel; when in the small intestine the area of pain is lower; whilst when in the colon it is lower still. The alarm points in acupuncture corresponding to these three viscera are also in the three reflex areas, which would seem to indicate that acupuncture, at least to some extent, depends upon these neural connections despite the fact that the true identity of the relationship was obscure to the Chinese. Acupuncture relies upon Head's Law to 'deceive' the body into responding to a slightly painful irritation on the skin done by acupuncture by sending out repair messages to the related organ. These areas of skins are known as dermatomes and this is described as one of the methods of selecting points in chapter 9. Some of the skin reflex areas are at a distance from the related organ, which is consistent with traditional acupuncture as well as modern medical thinking. It was an American investigator, Dr Janet Travell, who was the first Western medical scientist to describe the effects of stimulating these reflexes, although osteopaths and neuropaths had been making use of the principle for many years, probably dating back as far as 1874 when Dr Andrew Taylor Still first announced his new theories about disease and treatment.

It is now almost universally agreed that acupuncture works, at least partly, through the nervous system, but Dr Robert Becker, Professor of Orthopaedic Surgery at the Upstate Medical Center, New York State, USA, postulated a complete operational data transfer system in living organisms which controls such changes as growth, healing and biological cycles. He was led to this discovery by his successful regeneration of tissue in animals and the union of fractures in humans by the use of electricity. He claimed that this system was the precursor of the nervous system and interlocked with it to provide a link between the nervous system and the cells of the body. In a personal communication to Dr Margaret Patterson, published in her book *Addictions can be Cured*, Professor Becker wrote, 'I believe at this time I can unequivocally state that there are significant electrical correlations for approximately 50% of the acupuncture points. We have concluded, therefore, that acupuncture has a basis in reality. There is a previously undescribed system of data transmission additional to the nerves in living organisms. We believe that this system is primitive in nature, operates with an analogue type of D.C. electrical signals and is concerned with the sensing of injury and effecting its control of healing processes. We believe the system is located in the perineural cells and Schwann cells peripherally and the glia cells centrally. There is evidence at least in the glia that these cells are capable of controlling the operational level of the nerve cells themselves'.

CIRCULATORY THEORY

The effect of inserting the acupuncture needle is to cause either a constriction or a dilation of blood vessels, depending upon the particular points used. This is another theory to explain how acupuncture works; though it does not fully explain how this effect is brought about in the first place. However, we do also know that acupuncture can stimulate the production of such substances as histamine and kinins, both of which are thought to be vasodilators or, in other words, have the effect of causing an increase in the diameter of small blood vessels. Kinins also have an effect on muscular activity of the internal organs and lower blood pressure. On the other hand, acupuncture frequently has the effect of lowering the levels of these substances and, since they are well known to be potent causes of pain, this is another explanation for the pain-relieving effects of acupuncture.

THE GATE CONTROL THEORY

This is a theory to explain the pain control mechanism of acupuncture and was proposed by Melzack and Wall in 1965. According to this theory, the perception of pain is controlled by a mechanism in the nervous system which alters or modulates the impulse which will later be interpreted as pain. This mechanism is called the 'gate' and its function would appear to be some sort of monitoring of impulses which are going to end up as being registered as pain. If the gate is bombarded by too many impulses it closes and prevents some of the impulses from getting through. Now it is well known that the impulses which are interpreted as pain are carried by nerve fibres of narrow gauge called C fibres, whilst impulses transmitted by large diameter fibres are not interpreted as pain. Impulses from large diameter fibres have the effect of closing the gate whilst the small diameter fibres open it. It is thought that the acupuncture stimulates the large nerve fibres which close the gate and prevent the existing impulses travelling along the narrow fibres from reaching the brain.

THE MOTOR GATE THEORY

This theory explains the motor recovery effects of acupuncture in a similar way that the Gate Control theory is used to explain the relief of pain through acupuncture. According to the motor gate theory, there is a functional 'gate' which, when closed, prevents motor nerve impulses from reaching their target muscle. According to Jayasuriya the anterior horn cells (which initiate or relay the motor impulses) are, in many forms of paralysis, not dead but in a state of 'suspended animation' or 'hibernation'. In other words, the functional 'gate' is closed, probably as an initially protective mechanism to limit the damage from the disease. Acupuncture therapy, according to Dr Jayasuriya, sets up a heavy inward barrage at the motor gate which is capable of partly or completely opening it. This barrage of nerve impulses travels along the large diameter fibres in a direction contrary to normal. The full explanation of the neurological mechanisms involved is fairly complicated and beyond the scope of this book, but one of the factors contributing to motor recovery is almost certainly the activation of spindle cells. These tiny, elongated capsules situated along muscle fibres are made to 'fire' when the muscle is stretched. The important fact is that they are also stimulated by gamma motor neurons which are counterbalanced by alpha motor neurons, so that at any time the muscle can be maintained in a state of correct tone. If the gamma motor neurons are stimulated by acupuncture, the discharge causes the contraction of certain fibres known as intrafusal muscle fibres. This activates the spindle cells in the same way as muscle stretching. This ultimately reinforces the effect of the counterbalancing alpha neuron which brings about muscle contraction. The theory was first elaborated by Professor Jayasuriya in a paper read to the Fifth World Congress of Acupuncture in Tokyo, Japan, in 1977.

AUGMENTATION OF IMMUNITY

It has already been noted that acupuncture has an immune-enhancing action and this is brought about by a rise in white blood cells, an increase in gamma globulins and opsonins and a rise in antibody concentration.

Numerous other biochemical changes resulting from acupuncture have now been documented. These include hormones and prostaglandins which may account for respiratory improvement after acupuncture, serum triglycerides which may explain its effect on the cardio-vascular system, red blood cells which may account for improvement in cases of anaemia, and dopamine which may explain some of the results obtained in Parkinsonism and certain types of mental disorders. We are no nearer to understanding exactly how acupuncture brings about these biochemical changes, but the fact they occur has given acupuncture a scientific guise because its results can be quantified and measured by tests which are acceptable to any scientist.

NEUROTRANSMITTERS

Research carried out at the Shanghai Institute of Physiology by Professor Chang Hsiang-Tung and his colleagues have shown that serotonin and noradrenaline are also actively involved in the mechanism of acupuncture in pain relief. Serotonin is an important substance that plays a role in normal brain and nervous functioning. It is possible that serotonin is produced in the pineal gland, although this is not yet proved. It is certainly released in part of the brain known as the raphe nuclei and is active in the limbic system which may be described as the emotional centre of the brain. Other neurotransmitters are also influenced by acupuncture and partly explain its action.

ENDORPHIN THEORY

Endorphins are the body's own morphine-like substances which have the effect of abating pain. The endorphin theory is the most comprehensive of all the theories so far put forward to explain acupuncture in scientific terms. It all began with the discovery in 1965 of a substance known as beta-lipotropin by Dr C.H. Li and his colleagues at the University of California, San Francisco, USA. This was the forerunner of the discovery of opiate-like substances in the brain by John Hughes and Hans Kosterlitz at Aberdeen University in Scotland in 1974. The next year saw the isolation of two substances from a pig's brain by Hughes and Kosterlitz which they called enkephalins, from the Greek meaning 'from the head'. The enkephalins were shown to have a basic composition similar to beta-lipotropin and one of them, methionine-enkephalin (abbreviated to met-enkephalin), had opiate-like properties and was described as an endorphin which means, literally, a morphine-like substance from the body itself. This was a name proposed by Professor E. Simon of the New York Medical School, USA at a dinner hosted by the International Narcotic Research Club in May 1975.

The discovery of endorphins at long last explained the existence of morphine receptors in the brain, which could hardly have arrived there on the off chance that man would take an extract of the opium poppy. More importantly, it provided the much needed explanation for acupuncture just at the right moment! It was Professor Bruce Pomeranz of the University of Toronto, Canada, who first made the connection between endorphins and acupuncture. His primary interest had been with the field of drug addiction and he reasoned that withdrawal symptoms experienced by morphine and heroin addicts were due to the fact that the injecting of these drugs took up the receptor sites and left the body's own endorphins unoccupied. Because the body does not want too much of these substances freely moving around and having nothing useful to do it shuts off its own supply. As soon as the injections of external heroin are curtailed the body is deprived of its own source of opiates and enters a state of extreme discomfort. This is the well-known withdrawal state. Pomeranz suspected that endorphins might be involved in the production of analgesia by acupuncture. It had already been established that there was some chemical involved which was transported in the blood stream. This was discovered by administering acupuncture to a rabbit, connecting its blood supply to a non-acupunctured animal and finding that the latter now had its pain threshold elevated. The other two facts that convinced Pomeranz that he was on the right track were that mice whose pituitary glands had been removed could not have analgesia induced in them by acupuncture, thus proving that the chemical concerned was produced in the pituitary and, secondly, that the drug nalaxone negated the acupuncture analgesia. Since nalaxone is a well known morphine antagonist, this suggested that the analgesia induced by acupuncture was due to a morphine-like substance.

9 Moxibustion, Cupping and Massage

The word moxibustion is the Latinised derivation of the Japanese *moegusa* which is the herb *Artemisia vulgaris* (mugwort or Chinese wormwood). This is ignited and applied directly or indirectly to acupuncture points as a form of treatment. It is said that primitive people discovered the benefit of therapeutic heat accidentally by experiencing relief of symptoms whilst warming themselves by fire; hence it is a very ancient form of treatment, possibly antedating the use of needles. Even in prehistoric times they were practised together and this gave rise to the term 'acumoxy'. In Sri Lanka this is termed *vidum-pilissum*.

According to the Shanghai College of Traditional Medicine the heat from moxibustion 'Warms the *qi* and blood in the channels and is therefore useful in the treatment of disease and maintenance of health'. The herb itself is said to have a very *yang* quality and has the effect of regulating the *qi* and blood and expelling cold and dampness. When burned it penetrates the channels and is mostly used for chronic, weakened conditions where the channels have become obstructed by cold or dampness or for stimulating the movement of *qi* and blood.

The extent to which the inherent medicinal qualities of the herb are transmitted through moxibustion is still a matter of conjecture. Modern simulators of moxibustion which burn no herb but emanate radiant heat from an electrically activated sapphire head, or some other type of electrically operated heating element, seem to have good effect, though some acupuncturists hold that they are very much a second best to the real thing. However, the smoke emitted by the smouldering herb does have a physiological effect – particularly on the nervous system.

The herb *Artemisia vulgaris* is found growing wild throughout most of the Far East and much of Europe and this is a possible reason for its being chosen for moxibustion. The leaves are usually dried in the sun and rendered into a powdery form which is known as 'moxa punk'. Sometimes other dried herbs are mixed with the Artemisia. Different grades of moxa punk are available and selection is made according to the mode of application. The finer grades are used for making small cones which are burnt directly on the skin, whilst coarser grades are more suitable for making moxa sticks which are rather like large cigars and are burned at a distance from the point.

The following are the different ways in which moxibustion may be carried out:

1 DIRECT MOXIBUSTION

The moxa punk is moulded into small cones about the size of rice grains which are placed on the skin over the positions of the acupuncture points which are to be treated. Only one point is treated at a time and the moxa cone is ignited, preferably with an incense stick, and allowed to burn. If it is allowed to burn out completely, it results in a scar and this is termed 'Scarring Moxibustion'. The alternative method is to flick the cone off the skin as soon as any discomfort is felt by the patient and this procedure is usually repeated to a total of three or five cones at each locus. This method is known as 'Non Scarring Moxibustion' and is the method usually preferred nowadays, particularly in the West! However, Scarring Moxibustion has, apparently, been used successfully in the treatment of intractable allergic bronchial asthma in the People's Republic of China and the author has seen this used at an Ayurvedic research institute in Sri Lanka where it was employed with great success in the treatment of arthritis.

2 INDIRECT MOXIBUSTION

There are three main methods of indirect moxibustion: the use of cones placed over an intermediate substance, the application of moxa to the acupuncture needle, and the use of moxa sticks or rolls. When used in the indirect method, the cones may be slightly larger than when they are ignited directly on the skin. The following substances may be used as intermediaries:

a) *Ginger* A thin slice of ginger root about 2.54mm thick is used and the moxa cone is burnt on top of it. Very small holes may be pierced through the ginger. Care must be exercised to ensure that the heat is not so intense or prolonged as to cause blistering.

b) *Garlic* Garlic may be used instead of ginger and is particularly indicated for cases of chronic paralysis. Garlic may also be used as a heat transmitting agent over carbuncles, in which case the carbuncle is first covered with damp paper and the garlic applied to the area that first dries out from the heat of the underlying inflammation. The garlic should be about

½cm thick and replaced after five cones of moxa have been burned. When used in the treatment of paralysis it is sometimes allowed to heat up beyond the point of discomfort.

c) *Clay* This is made into a cake and used in the same way as the foregoing. It is recommended for eczema and some other skin problems. The treatment is usually continued until the patient experiences an inner warmth.

d) *Pepper* The powdered form of white pepper is made into a paste with flour and water and spread over the point to be treated in a layer about 2 mm thick. A slight hollow may be made in the centre which can be filled with a different herb such as powdered cinnamon or clove. The moxa cone is placed on the paste in the usual way and burned. The method is supposed to be good for arthritis and local numbness or stiffness.

e) *Salt* This method is used on the navel which is filled with salt to the level of the surrounding abdomen and this is then usually covered with a thin slice of ginger. The moxa cone is placed on the ginger and ignited. Sometimes, it is burned directly on the salt but in this case care must be taken to ensure that the skin is not burnt. The treatment is used for abdominal pain accompanied by diarrhoea or for general augmentation of energy and vitality.

f) *Other substances* These include bean-cake, aconite cake which may be made with yellow wine or water, or other herbs. None of them is currently in common use.

THE APPLICATION OF MOXA TO THE NEEDLE

This is a common method of applying moxa and may be done by wrapping moxa punk around the handle of the needle or chopping off a small section of a moxa roll, introducing a small hole through it and carefully fitting it on to the head of the needle. This, of course, has to be done after the needle has been inserted into the acupuncture point and therefore requires considerable dexterity to avoid inconveniencing the patient. In both these methods, the moxa is ignited, allowed to burn out completely and the process repeated two or three times. The needle should be allowed to cool between each operation. The second method is known as the 'OA' technique because it is particularly effective in many cases of osteoarthritis. It is usual to surround the base of the needle just at the level of the skin with a piece of foil or thick paper to protect the skin from any accidental dropping of the burning moxa from the handle. Needless to say, the practitioner is very careful during all types of moxibustion to ensure that the patient is not inadvertently burnt.

MOXIBUSTION WITH A MOXA STICK OR ROLL

This is the simplest method of applying moxibustion and may be done over parts of the body where other methods would be unsuitable, such as points which are covered by hair. The moxa roll is ignited and coaxed into a state where the end is glowing with heat. Again, there are several methods of practical application:

a) *Warm cauterization* The end of the moxa roll is held about 1 cm away from the skin and removed when the heat starts to become unbearable.

b) *Rotation method* This is similar to the previous method, except for the fact that the moxa roll is moved gently over a small area, such as the knee, which may require treatment. The moxa roll may also be alternated between two points, either in a continuous slow movement or by remaining over each point for a short while and then moving rapidly from one point to the other.

c) *Sparrow-peck cauterization* In this method the moxa roll is brought slowly to within a few millimetres of the skin and more rapidly withdrawn. The process is repeated until the patient begins to feel a degree of discomfort.

d) *Akabane method* This method was named after its Japanese exponent, Dr Kobei Akabane, roughly at the turn of the century. It is more often used as a diagnostic test than for treatment. A thin moxa stick or incense stick is used and the sparrow-peck cauterization method employed on the end points of the meridians (first or last points) which are situated by the nails of the fingers and toes. The joss-stick is brought within a millimetre of the point and repeated until a painful sensation is felt by the patient. The number of 'pecks' is carefully noted and each point compared for sensitivity. A point with greater sensitivity than its neighbours indicates a meridian that is out of order. The test is not used very much nowadays because the more sophisticated electrical diagnostic instruments called acupunctoscopes have largely replaced it.

3   THE HOT NEEDLE TECHNIQUE

Although not strictly moxibustion, this is another method of applying heat specifically to a point. It is a method which has been developed during the present century because, although of ancient origin, it was modernised during the Cultural Revolution. A special needle known as a *yuan-li* is used and this has already been described in chapter 7. The needle is heated in a flame until red hot and then thrust into the point with instantaneous withdrawal. It is particularly effective for benign swellings of the thyroid, other benign swellings, cysts and ganglions.

THE PURPOSE OF MOXIBUSTION

It is somewhat obvious to say that moxibustion is a form of heat treatment and that its purpose is to deliver heat to the body in order to achieve a therapeutic effect; yet that is a succinct, if not very profound summary of its purpose. Heat is well attested as beneficial for certain disorders and in 'ordinary' medicine is frequently applied for degenerative or 'cold' conditions. The precise physiological response of the body to heat has been well documented in textbooks of medicine and physiotherapy and may be summarised as an initial constriction of local blood vessels, followed by a dilation of these vessels which brings about an increase of the local blood supply in order to remove the heat. This tends to relieve pain, remove toxins and soothe nerves. In moxibustion the heat is more intense than that which is customarily applied in medical treatment, but it is also very much more specific and localised. Herein may lie part of the explanation for its efficacy because certain biologically active substances such as kinins and histamine are released into the tissue and these act as counter-irritants. The phenomenon of counter-irritation has long been employed in medicine and is the justification for the use of such medicaments as Spanish fly for the relief of pain. Roger Newman Turner and Royston Low say that it acts as a 'stressor' and they invoke the authority of Selye's concept of the General Adaptation Syndrome to better explain the effects of moxibustion. According to Selye, a stressor acting on the body elicits an 'alarm reaction' which, by activating the nervous system and the adrenal glands, leads to a 'stage of resistance'. Hormones produced by the adrenals have both anti-inflammatory and tissue healing effects and Newman Turner and Low say that, 'The initiation of a renewed General Adaptation Syndrome, by means of a target stressor at another site (moxibustion) reactivates the defensive mechanisms with a beneficial effect'. Evidence has also been adduced to indicate that other hormones are also produced as a result of moxibustion and that these include some from the pituitary. The Cooperative Research Group of Moxibustion of Jianxi Province, China, recorded various physiological parameters during and after moxibustion to the point *chihyin* which is situated at the outside corner at the base of the nail of the little toe. This point is treated when there is a malposition of the fetus. Moxibustion was found to have caused an increase in certain steroids without evidence of direct nervous stimulation and it was concluded that it worked by prompting the normal physiological process of hormone release by acting on the pituitary. The complete absence of such results when certain other points were treated with moxibustion leads to the conclusion that the point itself has a special relationship with the areas concerned and this reinforces the traditional belief correlating acupuncture meridians and points with specific tissues and functions.

In terms of Chinese Medicine, moxibustion is suited particularly for conditions of cold, dampness, deficient *qi* and stagnation. These correspond in Western terminology to such disorders as asthma, impotence, palpitations, oedema (retention of water in the tissues), poor circulation, loose stools, abdominal distension, feeling unduly cold, fear of the cold, kidney stones, tumours, withdrawn personality and diminished activity.

Moxibustion is forbidden at certain points and this is often for obvious reasons, such as in the case of points near the eyes. In the case of some of the traditionally forbidden points there seems no logical reason for the prohibition; although scarring moxibustion might cause trouble if it was done on the toes and would cause temporary disfigurement if done on the face or other commonly exposed parts. Some of the forbidden points are over superficial blood vessels and some are thought to be prohibited because of the strong effect that they can have on the body's energies. In general, moxibustion is not given to very young children, very old people, mentally disordered people, in diabetes, where there is a loss of feeling or anywhere near ulcers or inflamed areas. In all other cases moxibustion, if properly applied, is an extremely safe, comfortable and effective treatment either by itself or in conjunction with needling.

CUPPING

This is another very valuable traditional technique which also involves the use of heat, although in this case it is utilised to create a suction rather than to heat the tissues. A hollow vessel such as a glass jar or cup is used. In ancient times suction was applied to animal horns which had had their tips chopped off and were inverted over the area to be treated. Nowadays, elegant glass cups are made for the purpose and these may be attached to a vacuum machine. The traditional method of using the cups is, however, still preferred and is independent of modern technology – except for the manufacture of the cups. The doctor wraps a little cotton wool soaked in surgical spirit around a pair of forceps. This is ignited and introduced for a second or two into the cup and withdrawn. The cup is then immediately applied to the patient over the area to be treated. The rapid cooling of the air inside the cup creates a partial vacuum and flesh covered by the cup is raised into the cup. An alternative method is to ignite a small piece of wool infused with alcohol on a protected area of skin and invert the cup over this. The flame removes all the oxygen which creates a partial vacuum and produces a strong suction.

The cups are retained for about five to ten minutes, depending upon the patient, time of year, area being treated and the degree of suction induced. A strong suction can become very painful after only a few minutes. The cup, having been applied, may also be moved from one spot to another without breaking the seal. If this is to be done the mouth of the cup is usually lubricated beforehand. Cupping may also be combined with normal acupuncture in which event the cup is simply placed over the inserted needle. It may also be combined with a blood letting technique in which case a special needle is used to produce bleeding and the cup subsequently placed over the small incision to induce further bleeding.

Cupping is indicated in conditions of external damp invasions, stuck or congealed blood, stagnant *qi* and phlegm. These correspond to the Western descriptions of coughing with phlegm, chronic bronchitis, bronchial asthma, chronic back pain or lumbago, some types of headache and sprains. It should not be used in cases of fever, convulsions, inflammation, infectious diseases, over ulcers or abscesses, over hair or in very nervous or pregnant patients.

MASSAGE

Although massage has no direct connection with moxibustion or cupping it is considered here since it is the other traditional method of treating acupuncture points besides needling. Massage may be done by pressing on the acupuncture point which is known as 'acupressure' or may take the form of circular movements over the point with the finger tip. Traditionally a deep, centrifugal movement is said to disperse or sedate, whereas a light, centripetal movement has a toning effect. Pressure massage is normally done with the thumb, but may also be carried out using the palm, base of the hand, elbow, knuckles or fist. Rubbing, kneading, plucking, tapping, twisting, rolling and stretching techniques were also practised.

Apart from the general physiological effects of massage, which are improvement in circulation, normalising of nervous functioning, harmonising endocrine output, toning or relaxing muscles and improvement of digestion, there are also reflex effects which may be mediated via acupuncture points or by other reflex points or areas on the body which may or may not have been known to the ancient Chinese. A good example of these reflexes is that of foot reflexes described in foot reflexology or foot zone therapy (*see* Figure 10). This was certainly known to the Chinese and has merely been revived in the last hundred or so years in the West. The hand, too, is known to have reflex areas and the fingers are specifically related to organs or systems. The thumb is related to respiratory and liver function, the first finger corresponds to the function of assimilation and digestion, the middle finger reflects the circulation and heart function, the ring finger indicates the state of the nerves, whilst the little finger is linked with sexuality.

Reflex points are commonly treated by massage of one kind or another by osteopaths and some chiropractors and this undoubtedly contributes to the favourable results experienced by these practitioners. It is also an integral part of the therapy connected with applied kinesiology (*see* chapter 6) and many forms of 'bodywork'. Manipulations of joints is also part of the traditional massage employed in Chinese medicine and is sometimes called 'Chinese osteopathy'. This probably has the effect of breaking down adhesions, restoring full mobility, stretching contracted tissue and beneficially influencing the transmission of energy or *qi*. It may also enhance nerve function by releasing the causes of congestion in the tissue and impingement of blood supply.

10   *Some Case Histories*

In selecting a few cases to illustrate some of the principles and effects of acupuncture treatment care has been taken to provide as great a variety as possible whilst, at the same time, avoiding the selection of purely successful cases.

MR S.R., Age 77

This elderly man came for treatment for a pain in the right shoulder which radiated across the upper right side of the back and down the right arm. He complained that his fingers were sometimes affected with tingling or numbness. This problem had been with him intermittently for 15-20 years. In addition, he had been suffering for three years from a pain in the right buttock, which extended down the lateral side of his right leg as far as the knee. He also had acute gout. He had had his gall bladder removed seven years previously and was now on Indocid (a drug used in cases of inflammation, rheumatoid arthritis, gout and pain). Examination showed him to have a chronic underactivity of the stomach, wasting in the leg muscles, stiffness and pain in the right hip joint. He was diagnosed as having an obstruction of the circulation of *qi* and blood, known as a *bi* syndrome. This was thought to be the type known as *fixed bi*. Moxa with needling was applied to a point on the hip and electroacupuncture was given to points on the back. The leg and buttock pain (sciatica) responded immediately to the treatment. Needles were also given for the shoulder pain but this was very much slower to respond and never seemed to clear completely. The patient discontinued treatment, after only a few sessions, much improved but certainly not cured. In this case moxa was used to remove the dampness since this type of disorder is thought to be due to the invasion of damp which obstructs the channels.

MISS K.T., Age 19

This young lady complained of long-standing migraine which started as a pressure pain behind the eyes and radiated to the temples. Typically, there were prodromal symptoms of blurred vision and feeling 'vague' lasting for about half an hour before the onset of pain. Sometimes there would also be nausea which would start after the pain. She also complained of frequent 'ordinary' headaches and variable pain in the knees. The diagnosis was mainly an obstruction of *qi* in the gall bladder. A faulty ileocaecal valve was also diagnosed and corrected. The patient was found to have an allergy or intolerance to instant coffee and advised to withdraw this from her diet. This is quite a common problem and it is hard for many people to realise that such simple changes in diet can have dramatic effects upon health. This girl made a good recovery with four treatments.

MR M.B., Age 48

This man, who had a sedentary occupation, complained of impotence of several years' duration. Investigations found no organic cause, though questioning the patient indicated that it was not purely psychological as he reported that he never woke up with an erection. The tongue was pale and swollen and the pulse 'thready'. He was diagnosed as deficient kidney *yang* and given moxibustion to the point *guanyuan,* situated half way between the pubic bones and the navel. Acupuncture was done at the associated point for the kidney and at *taixi,* which is a point on the kidney meridian behind the inner ankle. *Baihui* was used to reinforce the treatment and to induce calmness. After five weekly treatments the patient reported a successful outcome.

MASTER T.N., Age 11

This young boy was an interesting case because he met me purely by chance whilst I was treating someone else. He told me he suffered from asthma and asked if anything could be done to help him. It was with some trepidation that I treated him without asking his parents' permission but it seemed that the opportunity would be lost if it was not taken immediately. Of course, acupuncture was out of the question, so acupressure was used, particularly the touch type described in applied kinesiology. The boy was told that if he wanted any further treatment he would have to have his parents' consent. The next morning, quite early, his mother was shouting down the telephone. I thought for a moment that I was about to be at the receiving end of a lot of criticism for treating a child without his parents' permission but was relieved and happy to hear her say that the previous night had been the first for ten years that the boy had slept without waking up with an asthma attack. The boy was given a few more treatments, including lasertherapy, after which he was completely free from his asthma. Unfortunately, when the mother subsequently visited the family doctor and he politely enquired about her son's health, she announced that he had been cured with acupuncture. The doctor then protested, 'Acupuncture can't cure asthma', whereupon Mrs N., a very forthright lady, said, 'Well it bloody well has,' and, as a final flourish, declared that she had more faith in 'that man than the whole of Queen Mary's Hospital!' Not exactly a piece of conversation calculated to endear acupuncture to the heart of a sceptical medical practitioner! Alas, for all her rantings, there was no further contact with either mother or child; though the boy was seen by chance four years later. He was still free of asthma but had become considerably overweight. The case has to be described as a failure since the 'magic bullet' was merely replaced by the 'magic touch' and no alteration to life style was ever considered.

MR S.B., Age 41

The problem here was osteoarthritis of the knee of traumatic origin and of several years' duration. The man was overweight, had frequent drinking bouts, lived on a very bad diet of predominantly tea, chips and white bread, smoked excessively and, amongst other things, suffered from schizophrenia. He was on regular medication to keep this illness under control, but inwardly rebelled against it, saying that deep down he wanted to return to his natural (schizophrenic) state. It was obvious to me that his poor nutrition, aggravated by overindulgence in alcohol and cigarettes, was partly responsible for his mental as well as his physical state but it was quite impossible to get him to make the slightest alteration to his life style. The most recent comment in his hospital notes made by the orthopaedic surgeon was, 'This man will be back within six months begging for an operation'. The man had asked me what I could do for him and in view of his refusal to cooperate he had to be told 'not much'. Nevertheless, with acupuncture, massage and foot-zone therapy, he was kept going for five years until we ran into trouble with the DHSS. On my advice he had stopped carrying heavy weights and had subsequently become unemployed. After much correspondence with the local authorities he had been placed on a government retraining scheme but due to his impetuous nature had not lasted as long as a day! Actually, from his description of what went on he could not really be blamed as it seems he was treated rather like a twelve-year old. The outcome of all this was that he was told that unless he had the recommended surgery he would have all his benefit cut off: a threat that scared him into agreement. He asked my advice which I was loathe to give so I prevaricated and told him that it was entirely up to him. He agreed in the end to have the operation subject to my willingness to continue treating him subsequently. The surgery was a failure and he was left in a far worse state than before the operation. At one stage his thigh muscles had wasted considerably and the hospital told him that it was because he was not doing the exercises which they had prescribed. The poor man had been doing his best, despite the fact that it was very painful and he was given some electrical stimulation for the muscles from me which, I told him, should be done by the hospital. Little did I realise that he was going to relate this statement to the superintendent physiotherapist who passed the message on to the surgeon who went into a fit of rage and told the patient that if he had anything more to do with me he would, 'wash his hands of him completely'. It seemed like a heaven-sent opportunity to retire from the scene – an opportunity I took without a second thought!

MR P.R., Age 68

Mr R. was a charming man who would probably not have complained if he was on his death bed. His main problem was high blood pressure due to deficient liver *yin*. He was treated with acupuncture to *ququan* at the knee and three ear points namely, liver, kidney and *shen men*. Special points on the ear for lowering blood pressure were introduced at the second visit. When the needles were removed the patient wondered if his ear might play a tune in the wind as he walked out of the surgery. He had a great sense of humour which I am sure aided his recovery. His blood pressure returned to within normal limits for a man of his age and the vertigo which he had also complained of disappeared completely.

MR K.C., Age 31

This young man's problem was psoriasis which occurred in a few discrete patches mainly on the arms and legs. In his case the technique of 'surrounding the dragon' was used, together with two or three other points. Surrounding the dragon consists of making shallow insertions with about five needles around the perimeter of the lesions. It is a variation of local treatment. It is often very effective and was so in this case. After about ten weekly treatments the lesions were almost gone and some had completely disappeared. A few more treatments at monthly intervals completed the process, but at this stage the technique of surrounding the dragon had been entirely replaced by *baihui*, (for calming and sedation), *hegu* (for elimination), *quchi* (for its powerful homoeostatic effect), *xuehai* (for its anti-allergic effect) and *lieque* (to stimulate the lungs which feed the skin).

MRS M.S., Age 52

This lady complained of insomnia due to cramp which occurred chiefly in the calf muscles. The points *houxi* on the hand and *neiguan* on the forearm were used as key points to activate the governor and *yin wei mo* which are helpful in spasms and cramps. In addition, they increase the activity of the parathyroid glands which help to maintain correct calcium levels in the blood. Cramps are often the result of lowered serum calcium levels. The point *yanglingquan* was used for its effect on muscles and tendons and, finally, the parathyroid point on the right ear was given a press needle. After one week and a single treatment no further cramps were being experienced and Mrs S. was sleeping through the night without waking. (The reason for using the right ear is, you may remember, because women are always right!)

MRS B.L., Age 58

This lady was smoking sixty cigarettes per day and, in the words of her friend, was 'Never seen without a cigarette in her mouth'. She asked if she could have acupuncture to stop her smoking and seemed like the most hopeless case imaginable. She had been smoking since the age of fifteen and in forty odd years had never been without the habit. Experience has shown that the most difficult smoking cases are women in the 25–45 age group who smoke less than twenty per day, but this case looked just like the proverbial exception. She was given acupuncture to the lung and addiction points in both ears which were electrically stimulated for twenty-five minutes. After the removal of the needles, a press needle was placed in the lung point of the right ear and the patient instructed to press on it at least three times per day and whenever she felt the urge to smoke. Not only did she never smoke again but, about six weeks later, when she brought a friend along for a similar treatment, she maintained that after the acupuncture she felt 'as though she had never smoked'. At that time she was feeling immeasurably fitter and was adamant that she would never return to the domination of Lady Nicotine.

MRS R.L., Age 56

This lady was suffering from severe post-operative pain after a total mastectomy undertaken for a malignancy. She had been enduring this pain for several months and was scarcely able to sleep at night or carry on a normal life. She was given acupuncture to local points and *hegu* on both sides, from which she obtained considerable relief. However, the pain returned after three days, though with less intensity. She was given a second treatment and a TENS (transcutaneous electroneural stimulation) instrument to take away and apply every day. She asked if she could use it more often and was told that she could. On some days she used it as often as three times but as the days passed by she needed it less and less. After three more weeks she was able to return the instrument but asked if she could purchase a new one in case the pain returned.

11 *New Methods of Treatment*

Since the Cultural Revolution in the People's Republic of China and the dissemination of acupuncture throughout the West, the application of modern technology to the ancient practice of acupuncture has been eagerly embraced both inside China and in the West. The close cooperation of traditionally trained physicians and Western trained doctors in China has been particularly fruitful in both introducing new technology and researching the effects of acupuncture in a controlled environment. Many acupuncturists in the West are unable to participate in this kind of research because they are shunned by authorities who control the means of carrying it out. Innumerable experiments which are virtually useless are regularly carried out at enormous public expense; yet vitally important research into 'natural' treatments which involve comparatively little cost are not even considered. Research which has a prospective and profitable end-product which can be sold by manufacturers excites the multi-national companies to sink vast sums into pharmacological development, but no company, even if it did happen to have an altruistic board of directors, is prepared to spend money when the probable outcome is not merely going to be a financial dead end, but would actually lead to a loss of exciting sales as needles, or other inexpensive items began to replace profitable drugs.

A new technique of needling called periosteal acupuncture was first described by Felix Mann in Britain and subsequently developed by several people, particularly Geoff Greenbaum in Australia. It is useful for painful conditions but in the author's opinion should only be used as a last resort.

The surgical suture embedding technique, whereby a piece of cat-gut about 1 cm long is introduced into the tissues, was developed in China during the 1965-70 Cultural Revolution period itself. This technique produces prolonged stimulation of the point or points and is useful in chronic cases of bronchitis, asthma, gastric or duodenal ulcers, impotence, low back pain and the chronic effects of diseases like poliomyelitis.

ELECTRO-ACUPUNCTURE

Francis in Philadelphia, Garratt in Boston and Oliver in Buffalo more or less simultaneously discovered the use of electricity for pain control in 1857-8. Francis used a galvanic current to induce analgesia for tooth extractions, Oliver used a direct current to alleviate dental pain, but later used an alternating current and went on to perform other types of surgery with electrical analgesia, and Garratt also used galvanism for dental pain and neuralgia. In Britain, Althus was the first to use this new technique and its popularity spread to mainland Europe. In the same year (1858) the College of Dental Surgeons convened a conference to investigate the technique and the members unanimously agreed that no local analgesic effect could be detected. However, one member, Purland, changed his mind after performing a successful dental extraction under electrical analgesia.

Since then, and particularly in the last twenty years, a great number of workers have reported both the analgesic and therapeutic effect of different kinds of electrical stimulation. The publication of the Gate Theory by Melzack and Wall (*see* chapter 8) stimulated even greater interest in electrical methods of bringing about pain relief. In China, doctors of acupuncture were already using electrical stimulation to replace manual manipulation of needles to induce analgesia for surgery and it was an article by James Reston, the journalist who accompanied President Nixon to China in 1971, that brought this to the attention of the West. Reston had an appendectomy, and was subsequently given electro-acupuncture for the relief of the post-operative pain. It was so successful that he was constrained to write an article about it and it was this article that was to change the face of Western medicine.

The first surgical operation to be carried out under acupuncture analgesia in China was a tonsillectomy in 1958 in Shanghai. Since then, almost every kind of major surgery has been undertaken under acupuncture; though it is generally agreed that it is not very successful for orthopaedic surgery. It is particularly recommended for abdominal surgery and for childbirth.

To obtain analgesia, a weak current of a few microamperes is used, generally in the form of a biphasic spike wave of a frequency ranging from 5-2,000 Hz. The higher frequencies are used for surgical analgesia, but lower frequencies are normally employed for routine acupuncture. Today, electro-acupuncture is extremely popular all over the world, including China, and there are many instruments of varying sizes and complexity which can be used for treatment, electro-analgesia for surgery and for testing purposes. For this, a probe is fitted to the appropriate outlet of the apparatus and is used to test an area of skin surface. When an acupuncture point is encountered, a dial on the instrument will indicate an elevated electrical conduction through the skin. A device is usually attached which emits a high pitched sound to coincide with finding the point. These instruments vary considerably in their accuracy and depend upon careful control of a number of variables such as pressure of the probe on the skin, relative dampness of the skin and emotional changes of the testee. It is very important that the operator is thoroughly conversant with the location of the points before attempting to use such an instrument. Its greatest value lies in the detection of points on the ear where they lie so close together that it is not difficult even for an experienced practitioner to needle the wrong point unless great care is taken.

Sometimes, electrical treatment for pain is carried out without acupuncture and the commonest form of this is TENS which refers to transcutaneous electro-neural stimulation. It was developed after the observations of Wall and Sweet in 1967, and Sweet and Wepsic in 1968, that pain could be relieved by stimulating peripheral nerves with an electric current. In Britain and North America this has become a recognised treatment by osteopaths, physiotherapists and chiropractors.

Sometimes the treatment is given without acknowledging its origin in acupuncture and sometimes the treatment is euphemistically described as electro-acupuncture without the needles! The only problem with this is that it may give the impression that acupuncture is being practised which may delude some patients into thinking that there is nothing more to this than a having an electric current passed through them. Moreover, if a patient thought that he had been receiving acupuncture he might mistakenly be deterred from seeking a treatment he really needs.

LIMITATIONS TO THE USE OF ELECTRO-ACUPUNCTURE

There are a number of contra-indications to the safe employment of electro-acupuncture as well as a number of special precautions to be taken. It should not be used on small children or very old persons, nor should it be used on any person who suffers from epilepsy or other convulsive states. It should not be used in mentally ill people, non-cooperative patients, or those with excess *yang* states. Patients suffering from fever or shock or who are restless and anxious should not normally be given electro-acupuncture.

There are some points which should not be stimulated with an electric current and the current should not normally be passed from one side of the body to the other. *Yin* and *yang* points should not be interconnected and it goes without saying that the current should be started at zero and increased

100

very cautiously. Ideally, a battery-operated instrument should be used so that there can be no possibility of a mains current passing through a patient.

LASER TREATMENT

In 1917, Albert Einstein first conceived the idea of laser, which is an acronym signifying Light Amplification by the Stimulated Emission of Radiation, although the technology to produce it was not at that time available.

In 1923, the Russian biologist Alexander Gurvich noticed that cell division in one culture stimulated a similar proliferation in an adjacent culture, despite there being no direct contact. He termed this process 'biological induction' and observed that the phenomenon was inhibited by a glass barrier, whereas a quartz one did not affect it. This led him to conclude that some electromagnetic energy in the ultraviolet range must be involved, since quartz freely allows the passage of ultraviolet radiation, but glass does not. The evidence that a few photons could induce biological activity gave rise to the idea that this form of radiation might be useful as a therapeutic tool.

By the late 1950s, Schawlow and Townes demonstrated the practical possibility of laser and, in 1963, Theodore Kaiman of the Hughes Aircraft Company, USA, made the first ruby laser.

It was accidentally discovered in Hungary that laser increased the supply of blood to wounds, burns and skin ulcers in both animals and humans. Studies in Sweden showed that laser can fortify damaged muscle and improve muscle tone and it was this that encouraged some beauticians to make use of laser on the face in the hope that it would remove wrinkles.

The specific qualities of laser are minimal divergence or coherence, which means that the light is in a beam that hardly spreads out at all; single wavelength or monochromatism, which means that it is an extremely pure light; and projectability over a long distance. There are various laser-producing materials including argon, carbon dioxide, gallium, helium, neon and ruby, but the optimal laser for acupuncture or therapy seems to be the helium-neon laser. This was first developed by Professor Inyushin and his colleagues at the Biophysical Institute of the Kazakhstan University in Alma Ata, USSR. The wavelength of this laser is 632 nm and it was demonstrated by Fritz Popp in Germany that the healthy human cell resonates at 620-700 nm; whilst the sick cell has a shorter wavelength. In rheumatoid arthritis, for example, it is 385 nm and in cancer it is 428 nm. Treatment with helium-neon laser helps to modify this resonance. 632 nm is also the wave length of oxygen and it would seem that this is another explanation of the particularly good effect of helium neon laser. Professor Rachishev, President of the Anatomical Institute of the University of Alma Ata, has coordinated laser research and, according to his findings, laser has been shown to be capable of promoting haematopoiesis (activation of bone marrow), assisting the regeneration of skin and damaged nerves, reducing pain and counteracting arthritis. It has also been shown to be capable of inactivating viruses.

Professor Plog investigated laser with a view to using it instead of the acupuncture needle, and the Mecherschmidt Co. in Munich developed the first helium-neon laser. Research in Alma Ata has also shown that acupuncture points are specific loci of energy exchange between the living organisms and the surrounding environment and that the application of laser to acupuncture points has unique advantages in treatment. The points are stimulated from a few seconds up to about a minute.

The laser may also be used for direct treatment of lesions and one of the most fascinating of such applications is its use in many kinds of eye disease where the laser beam is directed on to the eye itself, including the pupil and retina. Good results have been obtained in cases of iritis, conjunctivitis and cataract.

The use of laser in acupuncture or for therapy should not be confused with its application in surgery where it is employed for its heating and cutting effect. In this case a very much more high-powered beam is used. For acupuncture purposes it is 25 milliwatts or less and sometimes as little as 2 milliwatts. It may be used for virtually any condition for which acupuncture might be suitable, but Table 20 gives some of the conditions which respond most readily to laser.

Laser is particularly suitable for infants and children, or nervous people who are frightened of needles. The enormous interest in lasers is demonstrated by the fact that there are dozens of instruments now on the market and symposia are held several times a year on lasertherapy alone. The other type of laser most often used in acupuncture therapy is the infra-red laser which is particularly favoured by Dr Nogier and the French school. One limitation of this laser is that it is dangerous if directed on the eye. As far as their therapeutic value and effectiveness in stimulating acupuncture points is concerned the argument between proponents of each kind of laser continues unabated. Much more work needs to be done before we have a good understanding of lasertherapy, but in the meantime it appears to be a safe, effective and painless alternative to needles.

TABLE 20

Some conditions for which lasertherapy is suitable. Those marked* were internationally recommended as suitable for acupuncture treatment by the World Health Organisation at a session in Beijing in 1979.

Migraine and cephalalgia (headache)*
Trigeminal neuralgia*
Intercostal neuralgia*
Claudication (circulatory weakness)*
Ulcus cruris (leg ulcer)*
Menstrual disorders*
Duodenal ulcer*
Constipation
Hypertension
Epilepsy
Haemorrhoids
Diabetes
Irritability
Hives
Cataract
Conjunctivitis
Arthritis

Sinusitis*
Vertigo*
Hyperemesis (excessive vomiting)*
Bronchial asthma*
Colitis*
Insomnia*
Nervousness
Abnormal tiredness
Heart-burn
Overweight
Underweight
Nose-bleed
Iritis
Glaucoma
Emotional problems
Skin problems

CYMATICS

This is a treatment using mixed frequencies of audible sound which was developed by Peter Manners in Britain. According to his theory, the vibration or resonance of the cell is upset and this is what we term disease. By irradiating the cell with corrective frequencies, the harmonious resonance of the sick cells can be re-established. The instrument used in cymatics computerises the various frequencies which are recorded on a normal audio-tape. This is then played back through a vibrating head which is held against the area to be treated. As in the case of laser, it may be applied to acupuncture points or directly to the lesioned areas.

APPLIED KINESIOLOGY

This has already been described as a diagnostic method in chapter 6 but it may also be used for treatment. Strictly speaking, applied kinesiology is purely diagnostic but it has as it were appropriated to itself certain treatments which have been elaborated using the technique to evaluate them in the process. It uses a touch technique whereby the therapist merely connects pairs of acupuncture points by touching them simultaneously instead of inserting needles into them. It has also demonstrated that certain disorders of energy may interfere with the acupuncture treatment and are best corrected by simple procedures prior to any acupuncture. Many acupuncturists, however, regard these findings as speculative. Such disorders include lesions of the hyoid bone, imbalance in the body's ionisation plant which is connected with alternate breathing through right and left nostrils and disorders in the gait reflex which is connected with the neurological administration of muscular activity during normal walking.

MAGNETOTHERAPY

Magnetism has always fascinated man and it is probably one of the most elusive and least known types of energy which is currently scrutinised by science. It would appear that magnetism has a profound effect upon the development and health of both animals and man. The earth's magnetic field deflects low-energy cosmic rays which are the most prevalent of cosmic radiation and this probably changes at different parts of the earth's surface. Researchers have found that north pole magnetism has the effect of slowing down growth and producing nervous, fastidious and unhealthy animals, whilst south pole magnetism accelerates growth and produces animals which are dirty, aggressive and sexually promiscuous. A balance is what is always required but in disease states there may be an indication for either south or north pole magnetism. The application of magnetic poles to acupuncture points is still in the research stage but some interesting results have already been reported.

SONOPUNCTURE

This is a method of using ultrasonic vibration which is a standard treatment in physiotherapy. In acupuncture, an instrument is used which focusses the ultrasonic energy on to a very small area in a similar way to when it is used by dentists for descaling teeth. Good results have been reported by some practitioners who use this method but it is not a procedure that is thought by the author to be ideal.

ELECTRO-ACUPUNCTURE ACCORDING TO VOLL

The work of Dr Reinhart Voll is mentioned in the Appendix but it would not be right to complete this section without referring to this system. Voll plotted a complete system of acupuncture points and meridians on the body entirely by measuring the electrical conductivity. He found that this almost exactly coincided with the traditional acupuncture points and meridians; though he found an additional meridian which he claimed was related to the lymph system and he also discovered that certain points could be used as 'reference' points. By testing the electrical conductivity of these particular points Voll states that he can obtain an accurate diagnosis of the condition of all the systems and organs within the body. By treating the correct points with an electrical stimulation, the imbalances in the body can be corrected – often quite rapidly. The treatment is normally carried out by applying the current directly to the acupuncture points and needles are not used. This system of acupuncture is usually known as EAV.

AQUAPUNCTURE

This is a particular form of acupuncture in which a small volume of fluid, usually a vitamin solution or distilled water, is injected into the site of the acupuncture point. The rationale for this is that it stimulates the microcirculation.

MICROWAVE

There is virtually no limit to the imagination and a device which delivers a microwave impulse at the point of the acupuncture needles has now been manufactured in Australia and, according to reports, has been found to be very effective.

HOMOEOPUNCTURE

This is a clever combination of acupuncture and homoeopathy which has now been practised in Sri Lanka for several years. When a particular homoeopathic remedy is seen to be indicated it is administered to the patient at the tip of the acupuncture needle. This obviates the problem of the remedy being antidoted by being taken with a meal or too near a cup of coffee, etc. It is thought to be the best way that the remedy can be introduced into the body. Initial results appear to be very encouraging but it takes a long time to analyse a treatment where two different therapies are being administered together.

GINSENG

The inclusion of Chinese herbal therapy would be far beyond the scope of this book, but the use of ginseng has been so consistently and inextricably woven into Traditional Chinese Medicine that no treatise on acupuncture can be considered to be entirely complete without some mention of it. It is, of course, only in the West that the use of ginseng can be considered a new method of treatment. One of the reasons for its special place in Chinese medicine is that it assists and potentiates acupuncture treatment, probably through its favourable influence on the endocrine system and its ability to establish harmony and encourage homoeostasis;

It would be nonsense to claim that ginseng is a cure-all; yet there is scarcely an illness that cannot be helped by this herb. What is even more interesting and valuable is its proven ability to enhance health and prevent disease. It is, as it were, a general immunizer, and it is in this capacity that it is particularly in tune with the basic philosophy of Traditional Chinese Medicine.

The ginseng plant is only found growing wild in two small areas of the globe – on the rugged slopes of Manchuria and South Korea. So avid is the collection of this plant that it is doubtful if it can now be found at all, except in very small amounts in remote parts of Korea. Cultivated ginseng is found in China, Korea, Japan, Russia and USA. The best quality plant comes from Korea and can be recognised by the redness of the root after it has been steamed. Beware of the lucrative practice of passing off old, hardened carrots as top quality ginseng!

In 1968, Israel Brekhman, a Soviet scientist, found that an extract of ginseng improved Russian soldiers' performance in cross country running. He also established that experimental mice had their stamina increased by 35% in running and swimming tests after the administration of ginseng. Professor Petkov at the Sofia Institute of Specialised and Advanced Medical Training, after conducting many experiments with ginseng on humans and animals, concluded that it improves learning, memory and physical performance. Ginseng was taken by Russian astronauts to protect themselves from infections. It has also been shown to act favourably in blood sugar disturbances (particularly low blood sugar), in cases of inflammation, to protect against fatty deposits in the arteries (arteriosclerosis), to enhance the blood forming properties of the bone marrow, to improve immunity, to protect against harmful liver toxins such as carbon tetrachloride and alcohol and to protect against the harmful effects of X-rays. It also accelerates the synthesis of RNA and protein.

With almost magical properties, it is not surprising that many legends surround the origin of ginseng, just as they do that of acupuncture. One such legend from Kirin Province proclaims that the plant was born one summer night in the cedar forests when lightning struck a mountain stream. The stream was transformed into the ginseng root. Thus, all the elements of creation — fire, earth, metal, water and wood — are represented and balanced in the ginseng root, making it a veritable panacea for all illnesses.

EVOLITE

This is a therapy first used in 1981 by Dr D. Stäcker, Medical Director of St Joseph's Hospital, Bremerhaven in West Germany and Drs Andersson and Einarsson at the Departement of Surgery, Eksjöklinik, Eksjoe, Sweden. It was their contention that the biostimulatory effect of laser was due to its being polarised, and they found that a lamp emitting polarised light produced the same benefits as the laser. Its chief advantage over the laser seems to be that it is easier to apply and is more effective when used directly on lesions rather than acupuncture points. Research into the biochemical effects of evolite treatment has been carried out at Semmelweis University, Budapest, Hungary and preliminary results seem to indicate that it is a useful therapy.

12   *Pitfalls and Dangers*

Although acupuncture is an extremely safe form of treatment with no side effects, it would be more than surprising if such a potent therapy was entirely devoid of all risk. In the first place, needles must be sterile and, although this can be taken for granted when the treatment is done by a medical doctor or a properly qualified acupuncturist, it is surprising how much ignorance there is about what constitutes adequate sterility. Even if rigid sterilisation procedures are adhered to, it is possible for a needle to be misplaced unless priority is always given to ensuring that this does not occur.

Secondly, there are 'prohibited areas' such as the scalp of infants before the closure of the fontanelles, the nipples and breast tissue, the umbilicus and the external genitalia. However, moxibustion may be done at the umbilicus and Professor Jayasuiya in Sri Lanka and Dr Mohammed in Kenya have used points round the base of the penis in their treatment for impotence.

Next, there are the dangerous points which should only be treated by experienced acupuncturists. These are points around the eye, some points on the neck which lie over vital structures such as arteries, baroreceptors, mediastinum (chest wall) and spinal cord, points on the chest which are not protected by bone or cartilage, one point on the abdomen which lies over the gall bladder, points which are close to large blood vessels and any other points which lie close to vulnerable structures.

There are a few points, such as those at the tips of the fingers and toes and on the palms of the hand or soles of the feet, which are painful when needled. For this reason very fine needles are usually selected for those particular points as well as the face which is also rather sensitive.

Bleeding and bruising may occur at the site of the acupuncture and this can be annoying if it is on an exposed part of the body such as the face. Fortunately, it very seldom occurs but only a day or so ago one of my patients telephoned me as she was very worried because her thumb was bruised after acupuncture treatment. Massaging the point and applying some tincture of arnica ointment is the best treatment for this problem if it does occur.

A broken or stuck needle is a complication which the author has, fortunately, never encountered; though this does, apparently, happen occasionally. Never inserting needles beyond two-thirds of their length is the best precaution against this as needles, if they do break, usually do so at the junction of the handle and shaft. Repeated sterilisation tends to weaken the metal and for that reason needles should not be retained for a very long time.

The forgotten needle is something that worries every busy practitioner. Once when this was discussed by a group of senior acupuncturists none could declare that he was free from guilt in this respect. Although it has seldom happened in the author's practice, Murphy's Law had to ensure that it happened to the same patient twice!

FAINTING

If you are prone to fainting or are of a nervous disposition you should ensure that you are lying down if you have acupuncture treatment. As this is the normal practice in most Western countries fainting is not a frequent complication. It is said to be a good sign, however, as it indicates that the treatment is likely to be effective. One or two sitting patients have come over faint in the author's practice but this is an eventuality that can easily be dealt with. The needles are withdrawn and a special point for recovery is massaged.

ADDICTION TO ACUPUNCTURE

This is the only true side effect of acupuncture but it is both rare and harmless. It is scarcely ever seen when treatment has to be paid for and can therefore be described as a largely unaffordable luxury. One interesting case occurred in Sri Lanka where the patient would turn up from time to time and after careful appraisal of the situation would seek out the most incompetent doctor or student from whom he would solicit treatment. It seemed that the more painful the needle insertion the better it fulfilled his need!

WHEN YOU SHOULD NOT RECEIVE ACUPUNCTURE (OR WHEN CAUTION IS NECESSARY)

1 *If you suffer from any sort of malignancy.* This is because acupuncture is said to have no curative effect on malignant disorders. However, acupuncture treatment may be received for the secondary effects of the disease, such as pain, depression or insomnia. Despite this admonition it should be said that some cases of malignant growth have been successfully treated with acupuncture, including a nine month old baby in Sri Lanka

with a brain tumour which had been pronounced incurable. The infant was given six months to live and the mother, in desperation, had begged for him to be given acupuncture. When the author last saw him the child was doing fine and had already made considerable progress towards normal functioning.

2 *If you have a serious infection.* Antibiotics are normally the treatment of choice in such cases, although acupuncture may be combined with drug treatment. It may also be used if there is allergy or intolerance to the antibiotic.

3 *When surgery is required.* This includes those cases where accidents have resulted in dislocation or fracture of bones or injury to vital organs or blood vessels. Other cases for surgery include congenital malformations, mechanical obstructions or appendicitis. The latter condition has, however, been successfully treated by acupuncture in the People's Republic of China.

4 *During the first or last two months of pregnancy.* Problems associated with pregnancy are regularly treated with acupuncture but these months are to be avoided if possible. At all stages of pregnancy there are certain acupuncture points which are not used; neither is strong stimulation or electro-acupuncture given. Even this advice is only cautionary and the author himself recently gave very strong stimulation to one of these points during the last month of pregnancy. This was done with a view to getting a malpositioned foetus to turn. Unfortunately, although the treatment did cause considerable movement, the baby was unable to turn completely, but the outcome was a successful breech delivery.

5 *If you are taking medicinal drugs for certain types of illnesses.* These include diabetes, thyroid problems or high blood pressure where caution is required before acupuncture treatment as it may be necessary to adjust the dose of your drug in order to compensate for the effect of the acupuncture. In this eventuality it is highly desirable that the doctor who prescribed the drug should be involved in this process. If you take drugs for 'social' reasons or if you are under the influence of drugs or alcohol it is extremely important that you inform the acupuncturist before treatment. Acupuncture can be used to help you withdraw from such drugs but, in the last analysis, self determination is absolutely essential. The same thing is true for smoking as acupuncture can be very helpful if you want to stop, but it will not actually stop you.

13 *Finding a Practitioner*

The conditions for which acupuncture is worth considering as an alternative to conventional medicine are almost limitless. However, it should be fairly obvious that functional problems where there is no structural or organic change are much more likely to respond to treatment than degenerative conditions where organic changes have taken place. The prognosis depends also upon the length of time the problems have existed, the inherent vitality or healing power and the life style which may assist or militate against the healing process. In general, conditions such as headaches, migraine, hay fever, sinusitis, 'frozen' shoulder, 'tennis' elbow, early arthritis, asthma, vague aches and pains and blood pressure abnormalities respond more quickly and satisfactorily than long standing conditions where degenerative changes have taken place. Normally, in the West, acupuncture is not used for life threatening diseases for which antibiotics or surgery have become the accepted treatments, although in such cases acupuncture can constitute a valuable adjunct.

In childbirth acupuncture is particularly to be recommended, provided the full cooperation of the obstetrician and midwife can be obtained.

The following associations or organisations may be approached in order to find an acupuncture practitioner in your locality:

AUSTRALIA

Brisbane College of Traditional Acupuncture Ltd., 2nd Floor, Century House, 316 Adelaide Street, Brisbane, 4000, Queensland.

Acupuncture Association of Victoria, 126 Union Road, Surrey Hills, Victoria 3127.

Median Research Australia Pty Ltd., 128 Stuart Road, Warradale, South Australia 5046.

Acupuncture College of Australia, 520 Harris St, Ultimo, Sydney, New South Wales, Australia.

CAMEROON

Dr E. Emmanuel, Hôpital Laquintinie, BP 1041, Douala.

CANADA

Dr P.A. Gaulin, President, Canadian Acupuncture Association of Canada Inc. (CAAC), 512 Rideau Street, Ottawa, Ontario, K1N 5Z6.

The Canadian Acupuncture Foundation, Suite 302, 7321 Victoria Park Avenue, Markham, Ontario, L3R 2Z8.

EGYPT

Professor A.M. Radwan, Kasr El Ainy Faculty of Medicine, 16 Dr. Mahmoud Azmy Street, Zamalek, Cairo.

HONG KONG

Dr Tam Shut-Kui, 322-24 Nathan Road, Kowloon.

Dr Wing Kwong Tse, President, Chinese Acupuncture Research Society, PO Box 20088.

Dr Ching Chong Yan, 191-193 Gloucester Road, 8th Floor, Flat D.

INDIA

Dr A. Agraval, Indian Medical Acupuncture Association, Ramsagarpara, Raipur-492001.

Indian Academy of Acupuncture Science, Parli-Vaijnath Dist Beed, (M S).

JAPAN

Dr H.K. Nishihata, President, Japan Chinese Traditional Medicine Association, 34 8-4 Chome Yoshida, Higashi-Osaka City, 578.

Dr M. Konishida, President, Japan Acupuncture and Moxibustion Association, 17-1 3-Chome, Nishiogi Kila, Suginami-ku, Tokyo.

Kyola Pain Control Institute, 280-3 Shinyucho Takalsujisagura, Kawaramachi Shimagyoku, Kyola.

Dr Kazuya Yokayoma, Japan Society of Acupuncture, 44-14 Minamiotsuka 3-Chome, Toshima-ku, Tokyo 170.

Dr Osama Itoh, Japan Pia Extraordinary Meridian Therapy Society, Horikawa Building, 9-6 Higashigotanda 4-Chome, Shinagowa-ku, Tokyo.

KENYA

Dr A.H. Mohammed, City Hall Annexe 5th Floor, Mam-Ngina Street, Nairobi.

KOREA

Dr L. Chang-Soon, Director, Korea Acupuncture Association, PO Box 211, Seodaemun Post Office.

NORWAY

International College of Oriental Medicine, POB 9183, Vaterland, Oslo.

PAKISTAN

Dr Zaffar-Ul-Hassan, President, Association for the Promotion of Acupuncture, 7-Q/2 Pechs, Karachi.

Dr Mohammed Said, President, Hamdard Foundation, Nazimabad, Karachi 18.

PHILIPPINES

Dr Marquinez-Palanca, President, Philippine Acupuncture Association Inc., RM 509, Guido-Ver Building, Espana Cor. M. Jocson, Manila.

SRI LANKA

Professor A. Jayasuriya, Acupuncture Foundation of Sri Lanka, 28 International Buddhist Center Road, Colombo 6.

SWEDEN

Dr L. Berglov, Odengatan 621V, 11322 Stockholm.

TURKEY

Dr N. Ziyal, Bagdat Cad No 395/1, Suadiye, Istanbul.

UNITED ARAB EMIRATES

Dr Amr Mahmoud, Middle East Office, Ruwais Hospital, PO Box 3788, Abu Dhabi.

UNITED KINGDOM

Acumedic Centre, 101 Camden High Street, London NW3 7JN.

British Acupuncture Association & Register, 34 Alderney Street, London SW1V 4EU.

British College of Acupuncture, 8 Hunter Street, London WC1.

College of Traditional Chinese Acupuncture – U.K., Tao House, Queensway, Royal Leamington Spa, Warwickshire CV31 3LZ.

International College of Oriental Medicine UK Ltd, Green Hedges House, Green Hedges Avenue, East Grinstead, Sussex RH19 1DZ.

Register of Traditional Chinese Medicine, 18 Shenley Road, London SE5 8NN.

Traditional Acupuncture Society, 11 Grange Park, Stratford-upon-Avon, Warwickshire CV37 6XH.

USA

The Acupuncture Information Center, 127 East 69th Street, New York, NY 10021.

The American Academy for Auricular Medicine & Scientific Acupuncture, 1634 Gull Road, Suite 106, Kalamazoo, Michigan 49001.

The American Association of Acupuncture and Oriental Medicine, 50 Maple Place, Manhasset, New York 11030.

California Acupuncture College, 1933 Westwood Blvd, L.A., CA 90035.

Center for Chinese Medicine, 5266 E. Pomona Blvd, L.A., CA 90022.

Dr Willem H. Khoe, President, Acupuncture Research Institute, Spring Valley Health Center, 3880 S. Jones Blvd, Suite 214, Las Vegas, Nevada 89103.

The Institute for Advanced Research in Asian Science and Medicine, State University of New York, DMC (Box 124), 450 Clarson Ave, Brooklyn, NY 11203.

New England School of Acupuncture, 319 Arlington Street, Waterton, Massachusetts.

Oriental Healing Arts Center, 8820 South Sepulveda Blvd, Suite 205, Los Angeles, CA 90045.

USSR

Professor Foma G. Portnov, Piestatnes, 13, 229070, Jurmala, 4.

The British Acupuncture Association has overseas members in most countries of the world and enquiries may be made to the London office to obtain a local practitioner.

Appendix

Developments in Acupuncture in Other Countries

FRANCE

In both Britain and France acupuncture was known and written about as early as the seventeenth century, but the earliest recorded practitioner of acupuncture in France was Dr Louis Berlioz who reported the successful treatment of nervous diseases by this method in 1810. In 1929, Soulie de Morant, a retired diplomat who had served for many years as a Consul in China, wrote his famous treatise on Chinese medicine and used it to teach the subject to French doctors. Regrettably, when they had learned all they could from him, the French doctors took him to court and obtained an injunction preventing him from practising without a medical licence. Disillusioned by this act of treachery, Soulie de Morant became mentally disturbed and eventually committed suicide. His contribution to the progress of acupuncture in France will never be forgotten as it put that country ahead of the rest of Europe by about half a century. According to Dr Stanway, a French doctor by the name of Mauries has treated 108 different ailments exclusively with acupuncture under the critical observation of two other medical practitioners. Dr Darras in Paris has earned considerable fame for his research on acupuncture using thermography, though the foremost authority on this topic today is probably Dr Simon Strauss in Australia. Another world-famous development in acupuncture which took place in France is that of Nogier's auriculotherapy. (This is the treatment of the body by using points on the external ear.) Not only did Nogier map out an entire set of acupuncture points on the ear, but also developed his now famous auriculo-cardiac reflex, based upon his discovery that when a certain type of light is shone on a point on the ear needing treatment, a change could be felt at the radial pulse.

GERMANY

In 1690 Dr Englebert Kampfer was sent to Nagasaki in Japan by the Dutch West Indies Company and whilst he was there he learned the theory and practice of acupuncture. In the early eighteenth century he and Dr Siebolds introduced the subject to Germany. Dr Kampfer wrote a treatise on his experiences in the Orient which incorporated a great deal of Chinese medicine and acupuncture. The German Acupuncture Association was formed in 1937 and this publishes a widely circulated Journal of German Acupuncture.

Acupuncture was being used in Germany for the successful treatment of Parkinson's disease many years prior to the discovery of L dopa, the only drug known to be useful. This, however, does not include drug-induced Parkinsonism which is most often caused by the major tranquillizers, such as chlorpromazine (Largactil), and may respond to treatment with orphenadrine hydrochloride (Disipal).

Dr Gabriel Stux of Dusseldorf has undertaken a considerable amount of research in acupuncture and has successfully treated a great many conditions, especially migraine. Dr Reinhold Voll is world famous for his discovery of 'Acupuncture according to Voll' made by plotting points of low electrical conductivity on the body surface. Starting from scratch he rediscovered most of the traditional acupuncture points, plus a few others. By testing certain points which he terms 'reference points', Voll claims to be able to detect *scientifically* a disorder in its early stages, and long before it becomes evident by the manifestation of clinical symptoms. His plotting of the acupuncture points is very similar to the work done by Dr Nakatani in Japan and doctors in China who have quite independently shown the acupuncture points to be places of potential electrical transmission. Nakatani also discarded all preconceptions; yet, by plotting these points of low electrical resistance, likewise found that he had almost exactly replicated the ancient Chinese acupuncture points!

HOLLAND

The British College of Acupuncture set up a teaching institution in The Netherlands which subsequently became entirely autonomous. It has provided that country with a considerable number of very well trained practitioners. Medicina Alternativa, which is an international multidisciplinary medical association, and was the brain-child of Professor Jos Schade of Utrecht and a few other dedicated scientists, has its headquarters in The Netherlands. However, it has had its administrative offices in Colombo since Professor Jayasuriya assumed the Chairmanship.

116

Its first international symposium was held at the RAI Congress Centre in Amsterdam.

AUSTRIA

Acupuncture in Austria is entirely limited in practice to registered medical practitioners. One of the foremost authorities on acupuncture in that country is the Austrian surgeon, Johannes Bischkò, who filmed a Caesarean section, a dental extraction and the partial removal of a lung, all carried out under acupuncture in China, and showed them on German television.

HUNGARY AND CZECHOSLOVAKIA

In Hungary acupuncture has been used in a limited way and three doctors there have proved that numerous stomach ailments can be cured by the use of acupuncture. In Czechoslovakia, doctors have used acupuncture to treat muscular trauma, amongst other conditions. Although not so widely practised there as in many other European countries, acupuncture has already become sufficiently popular for an international congress to have been hosted there in February 1985.

OTHER EUROPEAN COUNTRIES

There are a few doctors practising acupuncture in Greece, Italy, Portugal, Spain, Turkey, Yugoslavia and Romania yet there is an increasing interest in acupuncture and other forms of 'alternative' medicine in most of these countries.

USA

The visit by President Nixon to China in 1972 was undoubtedly the major influence on the development and expansion of acupuncture in the USA. Several States have already set up examinations in acupuncture for licensing practitioners and professional organisations have mushroomed all over the country. California had more than 700 licensed practitioners in 1983 and it would seem that acupuncture is on the verge of receiving equal recognition with Western medicine in this country. Its fate may, however, be the same as that of osteopathy, namely to be taken over completely by orthodox medicine. A Private Member's Bill, which was introduced in 1984, would have more or less guaranteed that eventuality had it been successful.

USSR

In Soviet Russia, acupuncture has been taken very seriously and early in the twentieth century a research association in Oriental medicine was set up. Many Russian doctors went to China during the Second World War to study acupuncture but its practice in Russia did not really get under way until about 1957. Shortly after their visit to China three Russian physicists set up institutes of acupuncture in Moscow, Leningrad and Gorki. At the institute in Gorki, Dr Vogralik treated 250 patients with peptic ulcers, colitis, asthma, angina, endocrine disturbances, facial spasms and glaucoma. He obtained a 78 per cent cure rate, despite the fact that all the patients were failures of conventional medical treatment. Russian scientists have been at the forefront of the development of laser for acupuncture treatment (*see* chapter 11) and have also displayed considerable interest in the use of sound for therapeutic purposes. However, acupuncture remains relatively unavailable to the majority of the population of the USSR.

KOREA

Korea has an extremely long history of the practice of acupuncture, which is perhaps not surprising when it is remembered that for many centuries dating from 108 BC the country was considered to be part of China. Chinese medicine is thought to have been introduced to Korea around 541 AD at a time when its relationship with China was at its most intimate. In 1613 the King ordered the famous Korean physician Hsu Tsuen to condense and edit the material of seventy-two Chinese medical classics published since the second century BC. The result of this was Hsu's *Thesaurus of Oriental Medicine*. Hsu Tsuen was regarded as the Hippocrates of Korea. The first entirely Korean publication on acupuncture was produced in 1644 by another famous Korean physician, Hsu Jen, and was entitled *Proven Prescriptions in Acupuncture*.

In 1963, Dr Kim Bong-han, a professor at Pyongyang University, caused a sensation throughout the medical and scientific community when he announced that he had demonstrated the anatomical existence of acupuncture meridians. Unfortunately, his findings have never been properly replicated and his work has, at least for the time being, been discarded.

MALAYSIA

The progress of acupuncture in Malaysia is testified by the work of Professor Dr Kung Chieh, Professor Dr Wong Wai-Ming and Associate Professors Yu Chun-Ming and Chang Yen-Chiang of the Maktab Acupuncture Sabah

Malaysia, who have published their interesting work on eyelid repair with acupuncture. A good number of physicians practise day to day acupuncture in Malaysia.

VIETNAM

Like Korea, Vietnam has long enjoyed very close relations with China and historical records testify to the curing of the King of Vietnam of a serious illness by acupuncture in the fourteenth century. By 1403 the Vietnamese government had given official recognition to Chinese medicine by appointing a practitioner, Nyuen Ta-cheng, to be Minister of Public Health and Welfare. In recent years many Vietnamese refugees have brought their version of acupuncture to their host countries in the West and have thereby made a significant contribution to its progress and practice in the Occident.

SRI LANKA

Acupuncture is widely practised throughout Sri Lanka, thanks chiefly to the untiring efforts of Professor Anton Jayasuriya, who was sent on a WHO Fellowship to study acupuncture in China and, on his return to Sri Lanka, was appointed Consultant at a newly created Acupuncture Department at Colombo South Hospital. Hundreds of patients are treated daily and in the early years a large number of surgical operations were performed under acupuncture analgesia. Since then, an Institute has been formed and people from all over the world go there to learn acupuncture. In 1984, Jayasuriya received the Dag Hammerskjöld Award for Medicine.

OTHER COUNTRIES

Space prevents my dealing with every country separately as acupuncture is now practised almost everywhere. In India there are now a fair number of doctors practising acupuncture, many of whom have studied in Sri Lanka. In Pakistan a medical acupuncture society has recently been set up and is working to very high standards of practice. In Hong Kong, Taiwan and other Far Eastern countries it has been practised extensively for a long period of time and in the early days of acupuncture in the West, many doctors travelled to these countries to study the subject.

In China itself acupuncture has grown apace since the time of Mao. There are more than 3,000 hospitals and clinics, together with thirteen academies and hundreds of technical schools for the study and practice of traditional medicine and basic sciences. Their treatment of deaf mutes became world famous when Yang Fu-Chi carried out highly successful work on this problem by inserting a needle in the dangerous point of *yamen* at the nape of the neck to a depth not previously thought possible. Under the aegis of Chairman Hua Guo-Feng the first National Symposium of Acupuncture and Moxibustion was held in Beijing in June 1979 and the second in 1984. An abundance of scientific papers was in evidence at both of these symposia and even acupuncture practitioners have been amazed at the diversity of conditions which have now been categorically shown to be helped by acupuncture. These include leprosy, appendicitis, poliomyelitis, malignancies and type 'B' encephalitis: conditions which most European practitioners would probably prefer to treat with 'conventional' therapy! As it happens there is no such treatment for victims of the last of these diseases; in the West they are denied acupuncture and left to suffer!

Glossary

Acupuncture   Insertion of a needle into a predetermined and specific point on the body, with a view to enhancing the *qi* and improving the general state of health.

Acupuncture analgesia   Term referring to the elevation of pain threshold by the use of acupuncture.

Acupuncture point (acupoint)   Point of low electrical resistance on the body surface where the *qi* is capable of being influenced by various kinds of treatment, notably the insertion of a needle. The acupoints are probably loci where cosmic (electro-magnetic) energy is absorbed and eliminated by the body.

Ah shi point   A point on the surface of the body which is painful when pressed. These points arise spontaneously.

Alarm points   Also known as *mu* points, these are acupuncture points which are situated on the front of the body and often become sensitive during illness. Most meridians have only one such point.

Allopathy   System of medicine based upon curing disease by creating a different disease.

Associated affect points   These are a series of points found on the urinary bladder meridian which runs down the back each side of the spine. They are also known as *shu* points.

Ayurvedic Medicine   Indigenous medical systems found in most Oriental countries and which are based mainly on herbs.

Cupping   Procedure in which a vacuum is created over a small area of the body by the use of cups. Particularly helpful in cases of pain and congestion as it improves local blood supply.

Deqi   (Pronounced derchee). Sensation often felt by the patient when an acupuncture needle is inserted or manipulated.

Distal points   These are points which lie at the extremities of the body, below the elbows or knees. Their use reinforces the action of points near the other end of a meridian. Certain points are known to be very effective when employed in this manner.

DNA   Deoxyribonucleic acid. This is a substance that carries genetic information or memory.

Eight principles These are categories such as hot or cold, in which an illness or patient can be described.

Endocrine Glands which release their secretions into the body.

Endorphin Morphine-like substance which is generated within the body.

Five phases or transformations Sometimes known as the five elements, these phases refer to the cycle of life and are linked to the seasons, climate and emotions. They provide a useful framework for the interpretation and treatment of disease.

Gate Control Theory Theory which maintains that nerve impulses pass through a 'gate' which, if closed, prevents a sensation reaching the brain.

Governor The central meridian running up the back and over the head.

Homoeopathy System of medicine based upon the principle of producing another similar disease or diathesis.

Homoeopuncture Method of applying a minute dose of a homoeopathic remedy with acupuncture.

Homoeostasis Condition of equilibrium or harmony where everything is in balance.

Horary point A point on each main meridian which refers to the element to which that particular meridian is particularly related. It is a point which is usually treated at the two hour period when the meridian or organ is energised or depleted.

Hormone Chemical produced by endocrine glands which acts as a messenger to control other organs or tissues in the body.

Jing lo System of acupuncture meridians which permeate the entire body.

Junction points These are points on a meridian from which there are direct connections to the coupled meridians (e.g. colon and lung) or to the next meridian on the 24hr clock (e.g. colon joins stomach).

Ko cycle This is the control or inhibiting cycle which depicts the 'government' of one of the *zang fu* or organs over another.

Local points Acupuncture points which are situated over or around an area of pain or pathology.

Meridians These are lines joining acupuncture points which may or may not have a real physiological existence. It is said that the *qi* is transmitted primarily along the meridians.

Mother-son law States that the antecedent organ on the sheng or nourishing cycle is often the cause of a problem rather than the organ which appears to be affected.

Motor Gate Theory Similar to the Gate Control Theory but posits a 'gate' which prevents a motor impulse from reaching its target.

Moxibustion   Application of heat, traditionally by burning a dried herb, to an acupuncture point.

Mu points   See 'alarm points'.

Naturopathy   System of treatment based upon the principle that the body cures itself and only requires assistance in the form of natural or normal physiological factors.

Neurotransmitters   Chemicals, produced in the body, which carry impulses from one nerve to another.

Osteopathy   System of medicine based upon the principle that structure and function are intimately related and that disorder should be treated by correcting structural problems.

Qi   (Pronounced chee) Bioenergy or vital force which by its vibratory and spiral movements gives life to the body and maintains it in health.

Shu points   See 'associated affect points'.

Tao   (Pronounced dow) The unknowable Way by which all things are governed and which is expressed in creation by the two complementary forces *yin* and *yang*.

Xi cleft points   Sometimes called accumulation points, these are points on each meridian which are particularly useful in the treatment of an acute condition of the pertaining organ.

Yin and yang   Polarised energy which brings all things into existence and maintains them in harmony.

Yuan points   Also known as source points, these are points on each meridian which have a direct effect upon the pertaining organ.

Zang fu   Name given to the organs and their related functions in Chinese medicine.

Zymotic   Refers to fermenting process and therefore to diseases which are caused by bacteria which 'ferment' either in the body or in the environment.

Further Reading

Austin, Mary, *Acupuncture Therapy*, Turnstone, 1972.

Brodsky, Greg, *From Eden to Aquarius, The Book of Natural Healing*, Bantam, 1972.

Chang, Stephen Thomas, *The Complete Book of Acupuncture*, Celestial Arts, 1976.

Duke, Marc, *Acupuncture*, Constable & Co., 1973.

Lewith, G.T. and Lewith, N.R., *Modern Chinese Acupuncture*, Thorsons, 1980.

Mann, Felix, *Acupuncture, How it works and how it is used today*, Pan Books, 1985.

Meerun, Munsif, *Acupuncture Science and Art*, Mehar Printers, 1984.

Palos, Stephan, *The Chinese Art of Healing*, Bantam, 1972.

Rose-Neil, Sidney, *An Acupuncturist Visits China*, British Acupuncture Association, 1979.

Stanway, Andrew, *Alternative Medicine*, Penguin, 1982.

Turner, Roger Newman and Low, Royston, *The Principle and Practice of Moxibustion*, Thorsons, 1981.

Veith, Ilza, *The Yellow Emperor's Classic of Internal Medicine*, University of California Press, 1972.

Wallnöfer, Heinrich and Rottauscher Anna von, *Chinese Folk Medicine, Acupuncture*, White Lion Publishers, 1975.

Warren & Fishman, *Sexual Acupuncture and Acupressure*, Allen & Unwin.

Wood, D. & Lawson, J., *Five Elements of Acupuncture and Chinese Massage*, Health Science Press, 1965.

Wood, D. & Lawson, J., *Judo Revival Points*, Health Science Press, 1960.

Index